▶英語で学ぶ自然科学シリーズ 1
Introductory Series on Natural Sciences

英語で学ぶ医科学入門
Introduction to Medical Sciences and Practices

Ph.D. 渡邉 和男 編著
博士（薬学） 渡邉 高志
工学博士 王 碧昭 共著
博士（生物科学） 陳 佳欣

コロナ社

英語で学ぶ国際法学入門

「英語で学ぶ医科学入門（英語で学ぶ自然科学シリーズ1)」正誤表

頁	行	誤	正
7	6	to take	to be taken
9	13	10 seconds	10 seconds, (を追加)
11	下11	to take	to be taken
19	下1	divided in to	divided into
20	6	below in	below from
23	Notes:	1)〜5)は	1)〜6)は
58	6	er-ythrocite-	ery-throcyte-
89	2	extracelluar	extracellular
89	Notes:		extracellular matrix(ECM)「細胞外マトリクス」; matrices「細胞間質 (matrix) の複数形」
100	10	require and how	require how

最新の正誤表だコロナ社ホームページにある場合がございます。
下記URLにアクセスして「キーワード検索」に書名を入力して下さい。
http://www.coronasha.co.jp

①

Preface

　あらゆる科学技術分野での情報は，電子媒体を主体に容易にアクセスすることができる。一方，専門的な先端的科学技術情報を，正確にかつ迅速に理解することは容易ではない。そして，多くの有用な情報は，英語で大量に流通している。このような背景を考慮して，英語で学びながら特に自然科学分野での情報理解を支援するために，この「英語で学ぶ自然科学シリーズ」は企画された。

　編著者が1999年に執筆した「英語で学ぶ生物学」は，大学生の基礎学力支援を目指した教材としてのもくろみであった。幅広く生物学と生態学に関わるトピックスを紹介したものである。これが一般読者の利用も多数あることがわかり増刷りを重ねてきたことから，多様な読者からのフィードバックを参考に社会の関心や要求の高い分野を厳選して，本シリーズの展開を図ることになった。

　本書は，シリーズ第1作目であり，医科学分野を目指す高校生や大学生のみならず，一般読者が先端医科学情報に容易に接する手助けやきっかけになることを目指したものである。

　内容は，Unit AからUnit Eまでの5分野に大別されているが，オムニバス形式で，どの章から読みはじめても理解できるように構成されている。

　Unit Aでは，生活に身近な薬剤の使い方や開発について解説している。

　Unit Bでは，昨今急激に世界的な大問題になってきている感染症を取り扱い，Unit Cでは遺伝病関連のトピックスを取り入れている。

　Unit Dでは，医学と工学の融合分野である生体工学を主体に，今後の新しい技術を幅広く紹介している。

　最後のUnit Eでは，予防医学および医療と社会の関わりについて要点を論じた。特に最後の章で，自然科学としての医科学だけではなく，社会や人の尊厳を含めた議論を，生命倫理の課題としてあげている。

まだまだ多数の紹介すべき課題はあるが，本書をきっかけとして多岐にわたる著作を今後展開していきたいと考えている。

本書が医科学各分野のより専門的な英語学習への足掛かりとなることを願っている。

なお，本書の執筆担当・分担は以下のようになっている。

編著者
　渡邉和男
著　者（執筆者）
　渡邊高志　　Chapter 1, 2, 3（Chapter 14 は分担執筆）
　渡邉和男　　Chapter 4, 6, 7, 8（Chapter 15 と Chapter 16 は分担執筆）
　王　碧昭　　Chapter 5, 9, 10, 11, 12, 13
　陳　佳欣　　（Chapter 14, 15, 16 分担執筆）

2008 年 3 月

編著者　渡邉　和男

Contents

Unit A Pharmaceutical Science

Chapter 1 How to Use Drugs? ································ 1
Chapter 2 Why Does Drug Development Require
          Time and Money? ································ 17
Chapter 3 Are the Plant Materials as Both Medicines
          and Cosmetics Sufficient for? ···················· 32

Unit B Infectious Diseases

Chapter 4 Zoonosis ······································· 50
Chapter 5 Hope for Incurable Infection Diseases
          and Prevention: Malaria ························ 57

Unit C Genetic Disorders

Chapter 6 Dementious Disorders: Alzheimer's Disease ············ 62
Chapter 7 Chromosomal Disorders ···························· 68
Chapter 8 Hereditary Diseases and Gene Therapy ················ 75

Unit D Future in Multidisciplinary Medical Technology

Chapter 9   Cells, Totipotency and Organogenesis ················ 82
Chapter 10 Xeno-Transplanting and
           Substitutive Artificial Parts ···················· 88
Chapter 11 Nano-Medical Technology and
           Master-Mind Physicians' Skills ················· 94

Chapter 12 Machine-Aided System ·· 100

Chapter 13 Eyes for Blinds: Sensoring Systems ······························ 106

Unit E Preventive Medicine and Social Consideration

Chapter 14 Obesity and Exercise ·· 112

Chapter 15 Elderly Care ··· 122

Chapter 16 Medical Bioethics ·· 129

References ··· 141

Answers to Exercises ··· 144

Index ·· 165

Unit A Pharmaceutical Science

Chapter 1 How to Use Drugs?

1.1 What Should and Should Not be Taken with Drugs?

It has been believed for a long time that "drugs should be taken with water or warm water, not tea." What if taking drugs with milk or juice?

One reason for tabooing taking drugs with tea, is that tannin contained in tea and coffee (chemical binding of catechin and other substance) binds with iron contained in the iron tablet used for the treatment of anemia or a digestive enzyme-containing drug (e.g. amylase) and loses its efficacy. However, some of the recent studies suggest that the efficacy is attenuated by approximately 10 to 30 % and that there is no significant impact on the therapeutic effect. Other reason is adverse reactions of caffeine overdose such as palpitations or nausea seen when Over The Counter (OTC) cold remedies are taken with drinks containing caffeine. Caffeine (methylxanthine) is contained in many of the OTC cold remedies for the purpose of mitigating sleepiness, an adverse reaction induced by antihistaminic ingredient contained to alleviate running nose or nasal occlusion. This should be taken into consideration when taking OTC cold remedies.

In addition, caution should be taken when tetracycline antibiotics or iron tablets are taken with milk. Calcium and protein contained in milk bind with the ingredient and attenuate the effectiveness of the medicines. Meanwhile, laxatives should dissolve in the intestinal tract to secure its efficacy and therefore should not be taken with milk because they dissolve in the stomach before reaching the intestinal tract if being taken with milk.

Citrus is also included in what should not be taken with some of the drugs. Flavonoid, which has a blood pressure lowering action, is extracted from the surface of fruit and contains a bitter pigment flavonoid called naringenin. Naringin, which is, for instance, contained in grapefruit, inhibits the action of the cytochrome P450s, human liver enzymes decomposing drugs and xenobiotics. For this reason, the action of calcium antagonists (antihypertensive drug), caffeine and halcion (sedative drug), is reinforced if the drugs are taken with grapefruit. Carbonated beverages easily decompose aspirin (antipyretic and analgesic drug), which should be taken with water.

It is generally considered inappropriate to take drugs after taking alcohols. Drugs and alcohols are decomposed by the assistance of the liver and excreted into urine through blood. When drugs are taken with alcohol, alcohol is decomposed earlier than drugs and drugs are metabolized later, and this reinforces the action of drugs and prolongs the time when drugs remains effective as exemplified by declined clearance and extension of the half-life period. When being taken with alcohol, the action of oral hypoglycemic agents and insulin used for the treatment of diabetes is reinforced and may cause hypoglycemia, and this should be cautiously taken into consideration. Since cephem antibiotics and alcohol deterrents inhibit the action of the aldehyde-decomposing enzyme existing in human liver, concomitant intake with only a small amount of alcohol causes discomfort sensation. Concomitant intake of antipyretic and analgesic drugs, cold remedies and tranquilizers can cause adverse reactions and they should not be taken after drinking alcohol.

It is recommended to take drugs with warm water because hot

Table 1.1 Drug interaction and combination taboo

Medicine No.1	Medicine No.2	Interaction and clinical symptom	Measures method
interferon α	syosaiko-toh	stroma-related pneumonia	
ephedrine hydrochloride	catecholamines	caution required for the risk of arrhythmia or cardiac arrest	Reduce the dose and take cautiously.
three rounds system antidepressant four rounds system antidepressant	MAO repressor	occurrence of sweating, generalized convulsion, hyperthermia, coma, etc.	Avoid taking the drugs concomitantly and secure adequate intervals.
digoxin	Calcium injection agent	sudden manifestation of toxicity of digoxin	
sildenafil vardenafil	Nitric acid agent, NO grant agent (nitroglycerine, amyl nitrite, etc.)	reinforcement of hypotensive action	
β-spur (tulobuterol, salbutamol, carteolol)	Catecholamines (epinephrin, isoprenaline)	caution required for the risk of arrhythmia or cardiac arrest	
fluorouracil, anticancer agent	tegafur, gimeracil, theo uracil potassium	risk of serious hematological disorder	Avoid taking the drugs concomitantly and secure the 1-week or longer interval.
menatetrenone	warfarin potassium	possible attenuation of the efficacy of warfarin	

4　Unit A　Pharmaceutical Science

Table 1.2　Degree of incompatibility

\multicolumn{4}{c}{1) Absolute incompatibility}
Medicine No.1	Medicine No.2	State of incompatibility	Measures method
pepsin containing sucrose	NaHCO$_3$ Sodium Hydrogen Carbonate	activation of pepsin containing sucrose under strong acid	Pharmacists need to inquire to the prescribing doctor and recommend prescription change.
cyanocobalamin (Vitamin B$_{12}$)	ascorbic acid (Vitamin C)	100 % decomposition of cyanocobalamin within 1 hour (combination injection, room temperature, ph=7)	
meclofenoxate hydrochloride	lactated ringer's solution	rapid decomposition of meclofenoxate hydrochloride (combination injection, ph=8)	
\multicolumn{4}{c}{2) Modifiable incompatibility}
aspirin	NaHCO$_3$ sodium hydrogen carbonate	decomposition of aspirin	Pharmacists need to take technical measures in the dispensing procedure and increase awareness of patients.
levodopa	magnesium oxide	decomposition of levodopa	Pharmacists need to take technical measures in the dispensing procedure and increase awareness of patients.

Table 1.2 continuation

Medicine No.1	Medicine No.2	State of incompatibility	Measures method
trimethadione	ethosuximide powdered medicine	humidification and liquefaction after mixture	Pharmacists need to take technical measures in the dispensing procedure and increase awareness of patients.
trimethadione	ethotoin powdered medicine	humidification and liquefaction after mixture	Pharmacists need to take technical measures in the dispensing procedure and increase awareness of patients.
3) Tolerable incompatibility			
rheum powder	magnesium oxide powdered medicine	reddish discoloration after mixture	Combination may cause pharmacochemical changes but does not change drug efficacy. Sufficient explanations should be given to avoid raising anxiety of patients.
ammonia fennel spirit	seneca snakeroot syrup	yellowish discoloration after mixture	Same as the above

water may decompose enzyme preparations and because solubility of drugs decreases when they are taken with cold water. There are other various reasons. Some people take drugs without water but this should also be avoided. Drugs may stick to the esophagus and causes ulcer. It has been believed that drugs should not be taken with tea, but recent studies have revealed the effect of tea is minor.

Concomitant intake of multiple drugs prescribed by doctors, may cause pharmacological and pharmacochemical drug interactions as exemplified by discoloration or reinforcement of adverse reactions. Such changes are expressed by the term, incompatibility of drugs. Most of the drug information is the information about single drug. The following introduce changes of drug efficacies and pharmacochemical properties under combination or concomitant use of drugs for references (**Table 1.1, Table 1.2**).

Drugs have "expiration date" and manufacturers are required to show the expiration date if it comes within three years. Even unopened drugs kept in a proper place under the optimum conditions undergo changes in ingredient quality little by little every day. Drugs may lose their efficacy or even become harmful. Expired drugs must not be used and must be disposed. Once opened, drugs should be disposed in 2 to 3 months. Liquid drugs such as ophthalmic solutions should be consumed in 1 month.

1.2 What Time to be Taken: "Before meals," "Between meals" and "After meals" Mean?

When should the drug be taken whose bag a patient receives at the hospital or pharmacy instructs the patient to take the drug "after meals"? "After meals" is considered to mean "20 to 30 minutes after meals." Then, what is the reason for the time lag? The reason lies in the amount of secretion of gastric acid. After meals, a massive amount of highly acidic gastric juice is secreted and the amount of gastric acid reaches its peak in 1 to 2 hours after meals. Therefore, if the drug is taken in about 20 to 30 minutes, the risk of decomposition of the drug in the stomach is considered to increase. If the gastric wall is protected by the food residue which is still in the stomach, cold remedies and other drugs are absorbed in a favorable way without injuring the stomach. Therefore, drugs should be taken during such a time band. Taking drugs after meals is also considered to improve patient compliance. Vitamin A, D or E or other drugs absorbed after being dissolving in fat or digestive preparations which have direct actions on foods are also instructed to take "immediately after meals."

Then, what time does "before meals" mean? "Before meals" is considered to mean "30 minutes before meals." Then, what is the reason for the time lag? Appetite enhancers and gastric juice secretion promoters as well as antianginal drugs whose risk of attack after meal increases are instructed to take before meals in principle. Hypoglycemic drugs should also basically be taken before meals, but patients must never fail to take meals after taking hypoglycemic drugs which cause hypoglycemia if the patient does not have meals after taking hypoglycemic drugs, and patients must keep this in mind.

Some drugs, for example, antibiotics or asthma treatment drugs, which should be taken "at the interval of 6 or 8 hours" are instructed to take irrespective of meal intake because blood drug level must be maintained at the same level. When using such drugs, drug elimination parameters such as the total clearance[†] and biological half-life $(t_{1/2})$[†2], the time when blood drug level decreases to half should be also taken into consideration. Hypnotic drugs and drugs used to prevent nocturnal attack need to be taken "before going to bed."

Notes:
[†] total clearance
Parameter to show the ability to eliminate the drug from body (urinary excretion) systemic (total) clearance CL_{tot} refers to the total of renal clearance (CLR), hepatic clearance (CLH) and clearance by other organs.
(If the drug is eliminated mainly by the renal and hepatic routes, hepatic clearance (CLH) is shown as: $CL_{tot} = CLR + CLH$.)
It should be taken into consideration that urinary excretion rate

does not necessarily refer to urinary excretion rate of only the unchanged drug. In many cases, urinary recovery includes recovery of metabolites, and this should be carefully taken into consideration.

Urinary excretion rate of the unchanged drug gives useful information for the allocation of clearance to each organ. Renal clearance (CLR) can be calculated based on the systemic clearance (CL_{tot}) as follows. ($CLR = Ae \cdot CL_{tot}$).

Urinary excretion rate Ae [%] is shown as follows. $Ae \leq 0.3$ (drugs excreted by the hepatic route: $CL_{tot} = CLH$), $0.3 < Ae < 0.7$ (drugs excreted by renal and hepatic routes: $CL_{tot} = CLR + CLH$), $0.7 \leq Ae$ (drugs excreted by the renal route: $CL_{tot} = CLR$). Therefore, drugs of $Ae \leq 0.3$ (drugs excreted by the hepatic route) is less affected by the impairment of renal secretion which causes the decrease of renal clearance (CLR), but a decrease of hepatic clearance and systemic clearance will be seen in patients with cirrhosis or other hepatic disorders.

† 2 Biological half-life ($t_{1/2}$)

Parameter to show the speed of elimination of drugs from body.

Time necessary for systemic drug level or blood drug level to reach half when the administration of a drug does not involve the oral absorption process like intravenous injection or the effect of absorption is negligible when an adequate time has been passed after oral administration.

Measured data correlating to the speed of changes in blood drug level or systemic drug level is referred to as first-order rate process. Hepatic clearance (CLH) with elimination in the process is shown as follows: $t_{1/2} = 0.693/k_{el}$ (k_{el}: elimination rate constant: constant showing the elimination rate of drug via metabolism and excretion)

Then, what time does "between meals" mean? "Between meals" does not mean just between meals but is considered to mean "about 2 hours after meals." Then, what is the reason? Drugs which need to be taken when the stomach is empty such as those used for the protection of gastric wall such as antiulcerative drugs or drugs whose absorbability is low are generally instructed to take between meals. Herbal preparations are typical "between-meals" medications.

Antipyretic drugs or antiemetic drugs are sometimes administered as suppositories. Suppositories, which are easily inserted from anus, are used when the quick action is necessary vir direct absorption through the rectum. Cacao butter which dissolves at body temperature of humans is used as the base material of suppositories, and suppositories dissolve quickly and are absorbed through the rectum achieving the quick action.

Before concluding the chapter, I need to mention one more precaution. If a patient takes a drug while lying on bed or rests on bed immediately after taking a drug, the drug may stick to the bottom of throat or esophagus and this may cause inflammation or ulcer. Some researchers suggest that drugs act slowly by as long as 30 minutes when being taken while the patient rests on bed. Patients need to keep the upper body straight up at least when taking drugs which pass through the esophagus just in 10 seconds if they are taken with water.

As so far discussed, various drugs have various ways of intake depending on their ways of absorption. Patients may have not enough time to consider the optimal way of intake when they are sick or need to take the drug immediately, but it may be necessary to have information about how drugs are absorbed, transported and acted in order to ensure proper use of drugs.

Exercises

1. つぎの 1 ～ 44 の語に対応する英単語または英熟語を本文から選び出して書き込み，また発音しなさい（動詞は原形を記入しなさい）。

	Japanese	English		Japanese	English
1	タンニン		4	減じる	
2	カテキン		5	動悸	
3	貧血（症）		6	吐き気	

Unit A Pharmaceutical Science

	Japanese	English		Japanese	English
7	緩める		26	副作用	
8	緩和する		27	薬理学的	
9	鼻の		28	有効期限	
10	便秘薬		29	眼科の	
11	柑橘類		30	食前服用	
12	フラボノイド		31	食間服用	
13	ナリンゲニン		32	食後服用	
14	体外異物		33	服従	
15	拮抗剤		34	食欲	
16	鎮静剤		35	低血糖症	
17	解熱薬		36	喘息	
18	鎮痛薬		37	～に関係なく	
19	セフェム系抗生物質		38	催眠薬	
20	妨害物		39	夜間活動する	
21	随伴する		40	抗潰瘍剤	
22	(～のような)感じ		41	抗嘔吐薬, 制吐剤	
23	精神安定剤		42	座剤, 座薬	
24	食道		43	肛門	
25	潰瘍		44	達成できる, 到達できる	

Chapter 1　How to Use Drugs?　　11

2. つぎの各文が本文の内容と一致するものにはT(True), 一致しないものにはF(False)を, 文末の（　）に記入しなさい。

（1）The only reason for tabooing taking drugs with tea or coffee, is that tannin contained in tea and coffee, binds with iron in the tablet used for the treatment of anemia or a digestive enzyme-containing drug, and causes the attenuation of drug efficacy. (　)

（2）Attenuation of drug efficacy is seen when tetracycline antibiotics or iron tablets used for the treatment of anemia, are taken with milk because potassium and fat contained in milk, bind with the ingredient. (　)

（3）The risk of ADRs should be taken into consideration while using drugs. (　)

（4）In the case of being instructed on the drug bag to take the drug "after meals", it is considered desirable to take the drug in 1 to 2 hours after meals. (　)

（5）Vitamin A, D, E or other drugs absorbed after being dissolving in fat or digestive preparations which have direct actions on foods are also instructed to take immediately after meals. (　)

（6）Antipyretic drugs or antiemetic drugs are sometimes administered as suppositories. Suppositories are the dosage form enabling easy insertion from anus for sustenance of efficacy and rectal absorption. (　)

3. つぎの日本語の各文を（　）の中の語を用いて英語の文にしなさい（必要があれば単語を適切な形に変換しなさい）。

（1）水なしで薬を飲むと, 胃の中で薬が溶けにくくなるため, 効き目が遅くなる。さらに, 口の中や食道にくっついて炎症を起こすこともある。「コップ1杯の水で飲んでください」と薬剤師がいうのは, 単に飲みやすくするためではなく, 効きをよくするためである。(solve, inflame)

（2）貧血を改善するには，鉄分ばかり摂取していてはならない。十分な蛋白質が摂れていないと，赤血球の生産能力低下につながる。特に，ダイエットをすると蛋白質の多い肉や魚を控えてしまうため，鉄吸収のよいヘム鉄も不足し，二重に貧血の原因になる。(treat, cause)

（3）医者から処方される薬を「医療用医薬品」といい，その人の病状に合ったものが処方されるので効果が大きいが，副作用も強い。一方，私たちが普通に薬局などで買う薬は「一般用医薬品」といい，作用は比較的マイルドで副作用の危険も少なくなっている。これらはOTC薬ともいわれ「店頭販売」を意味する。(ethical drug, prescribe, risk)

（4）タバコの煙の中には，薬の効き目を強めたり，効き目の持続時間を短くしたりする成分が含まれている。したがって，治療期間中，そしてその前後の期間は禁煙をすることが大切である。(prolongs the time, reinforces the action of drug)

（5）薬事法の対象となる薬には「医薬品等適正広告基準」が設けられており，安易な広告は認められていない。しかし，ご承知のとおり，巷には『みるみる効果が…』とか『私も治った…』などなど，薬事法では決して認められていない宣伝文句が氾濫している。(medical supplies reasonable advertisement standard, admit)

Chapter 1   How to Use Drugs?

4. つぎの各問いに英語で答えなさい。

(1) Why don't you take medicines with tea, and you had better take the medicines with water or tepid water, if you can do it?

(2) May patient take a tablet and a capsule without water?

(3) Will unopened medicines be all right to be taken, even if medicines were past a time limit?

(4) Why you can't rub ointment when you have the inflammation of rash?

(5) Will it true that there are medicines that you had better to take with milk?

(6) Why a patient had better to take medicines on proper standing position than he lays down?

Reference: What is RCJ Pictogram?

To support good medication compliance, RCJ developed pictograms on "How to use", "When to take", "Precautions" and several others, that are comprehensible at a glance for everyone regardless of age. Pharmacists are recommended to use Pictograms to reinforce the patient instruction. They can help prevent missed doses and wrong doses.

—— How? ——

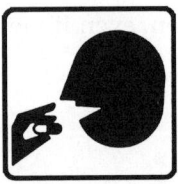
Internal Medicine
(Take orally.)

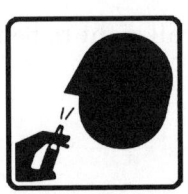
Nasal drops
(Insert the dispenser into a nostril and nebulize into the nasal cavity.)

Inhalant
(Nebulize into throat.)

Suppository
(Insert into the anus.)

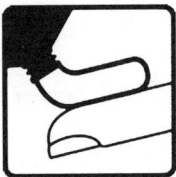
Ointment
(Apply to the skin, etc.)

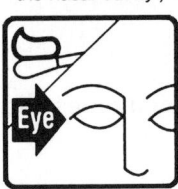
Eye Ointment
(Apply to the surface of the eye.)

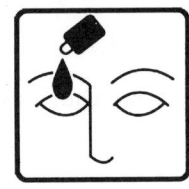
Eye drops
(Apply to the eyes.)

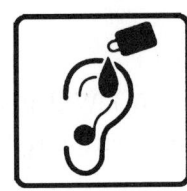
Eardrops
(Apply to the ears.)

Sublingual Tablet
(Dissolve under the tongue.)

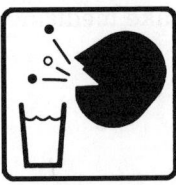
Mouthwash
(Gargle to use.)

Liquid Medicine
(Medicine in liquid form.)

Chapter 1   How to Use Drugs?   **15**

—— When? ——

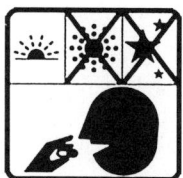 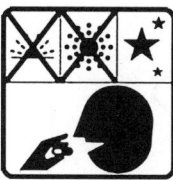 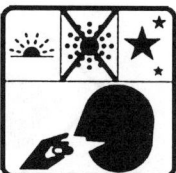 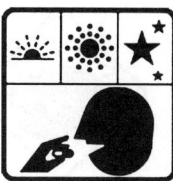

Take once in the morning.   Take once at night.   Take twice daily, in the morning and at night.   Take 3 times daily, in the morning, afternoon, and at night.

   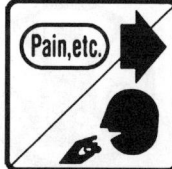

Eat 30 minutes after taking.   Wait 30 minutes after eating.   Take between meals.   Take only when symptoms appear.

—— Precautions ——

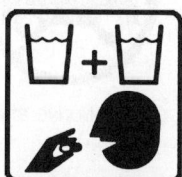  

Take with plenty of water.   Shake well before use.   Take at night before bed.

 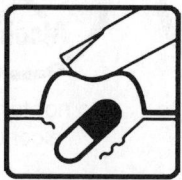 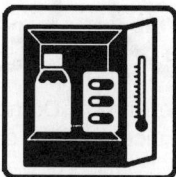

Wash hands before and after applying.   Remove the capsule from its package.   Refrigerate.

In your daily life

May cause dizziness.

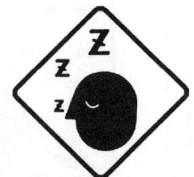
May cause drowsiness.

Prohibition

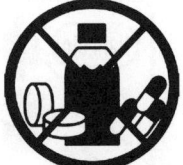
Never take with other medications.

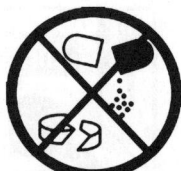
Do not break the tablet or capsule.

Keep out of reach of children.

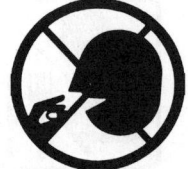
Do not ingest.

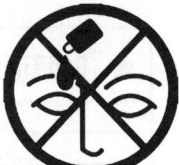
Do not apply to the eyes.

Do not take before sleeping.

Do not shake a bottle.

Do not drive after use.

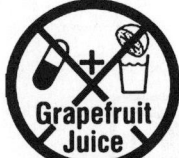
Do not take with grapefruit juice.

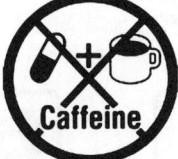
Do not take with caffeine.

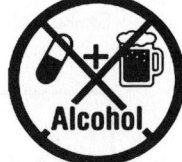
Do not take with alcohol.

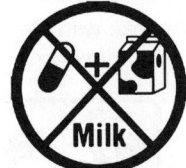
Do not take with milk.

(produced by RAD-AR (Risk / Benefit Assessment of Drugs—Analysis & Response) Council, Japan)

Chapter 2   Why Does Drug Development Require Time and Money?

Drugs are defined to be the "substances used for the diagnosis, treatment or prevention of diseases in humans." Therefore, people engaged in drug development have to be aware of the supreme goal of promoting the health of people and contributing to the future of healthcare. Drugs are considered to involve three factors as basic characteristics: 1) "biological action" effective for living body, 2) physically and chemically defined "physical properties" and 3) goods with "economic nature" having social functions and exchangeable values. Recently, however, the fourth factor, "reasonability" required for healthcare-related article, has been added to the existing properties as a result that drug safety attracts public attention than before. To introduce drugs satisfying these four factors to the market, the chemical compound needs to be not only effective but satisfy various factors such as safety requirements, pharmacokinetic requirements (absorption-distribution-metabolism-excretion), physical requirements, manufacturing-and supply-related requirements, economic requirements and patent-related requirements. Therefore, it is unavoidable that drug development needs a huge amount of money.

It is necessary to have at least 15 years before a drug becomes available on the market. Specifically, more than a decade and the advanced investment amounting to almost 20 billion yen are spent per product at the stage of research and development. Drugs undergo various complicated steps before they are launched (**Figure 2.1**). Research and development of drugs needs long and diversified

Notes:

treatment or prevention of diseases「治療または予防」, drug development「創薬」

Unit A Pharmaceutical Science

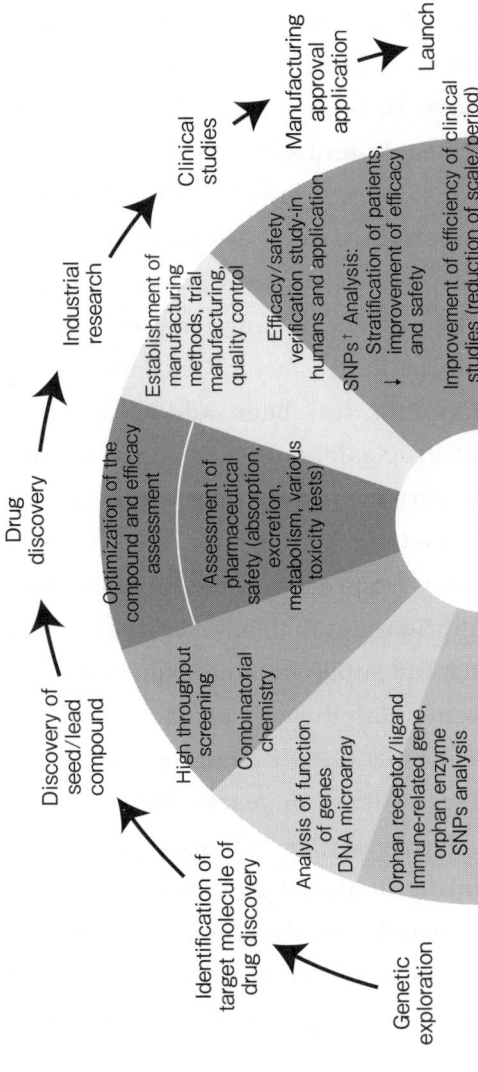

† SNPs: Single nucleotide polymorphism; SNPs refer to the difference of one base in the base sequence of genome. SNPs is related to individual differences in predispositions and is considered applicable to the exploration of disease-related gene, pathological risk diagnosis or response/ADRs to drugs.

Figure 2.1 Processes before launch of a new drug (Exhibition: Takeda Pharmaceutical Co., Ltd. http://www.takeda/co.jp/r-d/development/index.html)

researches. During the period, drug development may encounter premature abortion as a result of the advancement of medicine with respect to the safety or efficacy of drugs or changes of pathological trend or medical diagnostic criteria. Therefore, despite the investment of a huge amount of development cost, the percentage of successful development is extremely low compared to the development in other areas and the risk of drug development is high. The percentage of approval of a product item to all synthetic compounds is about 1 in 10,000.

Recently, Japan, the U.S. and Europe are all concerned with escalating medical expenses. In particular, in Japan where falling of birth rate and aging of population are remarkable, the government is adopting the policies to streamline the health insurance budget and cut medical expenses including constant lowering of drug price (price of healthcare products). On the other hand, as a result of the renovation and advancement of drug discovery procedures, manufacturers are required to obtain efficacy, safety and quality data at a higher level and these also boost R&D costs. It is reported that total costs spent are about 80 to 100 billion yen to develop one product in the average covering unsuccessful developments. For this reason, drugs are priced high to absorb a huge amount of R&D costs when new drugs are launched.

2.1 Before Markets

In this paragraph, I will explain the processes a drug undergoes before it is launched to the market.

The process is roughly divided in to 1) the stage of determining

---

Note :
falling of birth rate 「少子化」

the theme for the research and development of the drug (planning) and 2) stages after the discovery of the drug candidate (development). The former planning stage refers to the stage of development planning in which the potential of the research and drug is reviewed without the specific picture from a product. In the practical procedures, factors are described below in i) to vi) are reviewed, forecasted, assessed and planned. i) Healthcare needs: The trend of the disease, the situation of the society and demographic composition, availability of drugs indicated for various diseases and the social insurance system and drug pricing system are assessed. ii) Marketability: The profitability for investment is assessed. iii) Scientific and technological standard: The degree of advancement of basic researches and researches performed to identify the causes of diseases, diagnostic methods, target substances and screening methods via information from literature and scientific journals are assessed. iv) Percentage of success: The degree of difficulty of the development (judged from the scientific and technological standard in iii) or clinical study method) is determined. v) Competitiveness of the company: The R&D competence, sales ability, human and financial resources, availability of the company product, necessity and possibility of co-development and the range of development (acceptability of overseas advancement) are assessed. vi) R&D trend: The priority of development is decided based on the investigation of the presence or absence of internal competing projects. The patent application status is also investigated. As so far discussed, at the stage of development planning, manufacturers need to perform diversified surveys and objective analyses.

On the other hand, the latter stage refers to a more specific and advanced stage. The results of assessment at the stage of development planning are often subject to review and correction along with the passage of time and change of the situation. At a more specific

Chapter 2   Why Does Drug Development Require Time and Money?   21

stage, all departments are involved in the development, i.e. departments engaged in R&D, planning, sales, production and intellectual property (patent), participate in the development planning.

2.2   Non-clinical and Clinical Studies

As mentioned later, the next development stage is divided into non-clinical studies performed using animals and clinical studies performed in humans.

2.2.1   Non-clinical studies

At the stage of non-clinical studies, studies and assessments are described below from i) to v) need to be performed for the candidate compound.

　　i) Animal experiments are performed to assess drug efficacy, safety (acute toxicity, subacute toxicity, chronic toxicity, specific toxicity), pharmacokinetic (absorption, distribution, metabolism, excretion) and general pharmacology.

　　ii) Assessment of manufacturing/distribution: The feasibility of manufacturing and distributing chemical compounds meeting a certain quality standard in compliance with GLP (good laboratory practice), GCP (good clinical practice) and GMP (good manufacturing practice), manufacturing costs and manufacturing methods based on the consideration for safety and environmental effects are assessed.

　　iii) Assessment of physical/safety properties, iv) Assessment of formulation technique, and v) Assessment of clinical study analysis

Notes :
GLP (good laboratory practice)「医薬品安全性試験実施基準」
GCP (good clinical practice)「臨床試験実施に関する基準」
GMP (good manufacturing practice)「医薬品製造管理および品質管理基準」

methods.

For the above mentioned five items, protocols and schedules are established. If all data satisfy a certain standard, the manufacturer can advance to the stage of clinical studies in humans (clinical trials).

2.2.2 Clinical studies

At the stage of clinical studies, i) study protocol, ii) method of clinical evaluation and endpoint, iii) schedule and expenses for clinical studies and drug approval application and iv) development plan for Japan/U.S./Europe (An increasing number of products are developed in Japan/U.S./Europe under global strategies since mutual acceptance of foreign clinical study data was agreed and these data was allowed to be used as new drug approval application materials in other countries) are assessed.

Development based on relatively high leveled analytical chemistry is considered necessarily to perform a basic research about quality control or safety before performing toxicological or clinical assessments of a new drug candidate. The criteria of being the drug substance is established and techniques to assess a large amount of the drug substance and the developed finial preparation are devised. Chemical, physical and biological specifications of the drug candidate are tentatively established. If a chemical compound is demonstrated to have a favorable activity in the experiment system and safe in the toxicity studies, the chemical compound is a candidate substance (drug) for the clinical studies. Therefore, the first clinical study of a drug substance in humans is performed with strict caution under restricted conditions. Studies called Phase I are performed to verify the safety in humans. If the restriction is demonstrated and satisfied, the drug substance is assessed by the specialists performing Phase II studies, which determine the efficacy for the patients. After Phase II

Chapter 2 Why Does Drug Development Require Time and Money?

studies, the anticipated usability of the drug substance is guaranteed, the drug substance is more widely distributed to the investigators (clinicians) assigned to be engaged in the Phase III studies. At this stage, the studies are performed for the purpose of collecting data regarding the efficacy of the drug substance and the incidence of ADRs (side effects) from a large number of patient populations.

The modern history of drugs is the history of drug disaster. No drug is free from ADRs. ADRs may sometimes fatal and measures against ADRs are the important challenges of healthcare professionals. Before and after the world wars, drug disasters such as the case of fatal penicillin shock[1]†, thalidomide case[2], accident caused by the cold remedy ampoule[3], SMON case[4], chloroquine retinopathy[5] and sorivudine case[6] have cast shadow on the society. As part of the improvement of the system for compensating victims of drug disaster, various frameworks have been enforced for checking the processes to manufacturing, approval and launch (Phases I to IV) (**Figure 2.2**).

---

2 to 3 years
  Exploration of the target molecule
  For instance, target molecule receptor or enzyme is explored and identified based on the mechanism of development of the disease.
  ↓

  Exploration of the hit compound
  For instance, a drug substance reacting with the target molecule is screened using the automatic high throughput

---

Figure 2.2 R and D flow toward drug commercialization

Notes:
† 1)〜5)は 25 〜 27 ページの解説を参照。
chloroquine retinopathy「クロロキン網膜症」

system to discover the drug seed mainly from the library of compounds produced from natural herbal resources.

⬇

Designing and optimization of the lead compound

For instance, the candidate compound most appropriate for a drug is selected through chemical modification based on efficacy, pharmacokinetic, safety and stability parameters.

⬇

3 to 5 years

Non-clinical studies (including drug discovery to industrialization researches)

Animal experiments are performed to assess efficacy, pharmacokinetics and safety of the candidate compound. Physical and pharmaceutical tests are also performed.

⬇

3 to 7 years

Clinical studies (Phases I to III)

Clinical studies are performed in humans to assess efficacy and safety and the dosage and administration are decided.

⬇

1 to 2 years

Approval application

Nonclinical study data and clinical study data are summarized and the application for approval of manufacturing and distribution is submitted to MHLW using the designated document form.

⬇

4 to 6 years

Approval/marketing

Through the strict review by Pharmaceuticals and Medical Devices Agency (PMDA) and based on the recommendation by Regulatory Affairs Council (currently named Regulatory Affairs and Food Sanitation Council (RAFSC)), the Minister of Health, Labor and Welfare grants approval.

Figure 2.2 continuation (1)

>
> Post-marketing clinical study (Phase IV)
> The post-marketing clinical study refers to the useful study performed supplementally after manufacturing approval is granted to assess specifics which can not be assessed in clinical trials such as concomitant use, age or gender difference in a larger number of patient populations.

Figure 2.2 continuation (2)

1) Penicillin was an innovative drug developed in the age without antibiotics. Because it was drastically effective for infections, a drug myth that penicillin was a miracle drug that would cure previously fatal diseases was created. However, an accident which warned against overconfidence in drugs took place. In 1956, a patient developed allergy reaction with severe shock called anaphylactic shock after receiving an injection of penicillin during the treatment of dental caries, fell into coma and died after being admitted to a hospital in Tokyo.

2) Thalidomide was a hypnotic drug developed by old West German pharmaceutical company Grünenthal. The drug was originally developed as anticonvulsion drug for epileptic patients. In around 1960, the tragic evet that pregnant women who used thalidomide gave birth to children with deformity of extremities called phocomelia took place. Thalidomide was used as an antiemetic to combat morning sickness. The case spread not only in West Germany but many countries including Japan. Since Dr. W. Lenz, Hambourg University pointed out the relation between thalidomide and deformities of extremities in the Congress of Rhine Westphalia Pediatricians, drugs containing thalidomide were completely recalled.

3) Ampoule cold remedies refer to liquid antipyretic and analgesic preparations containing aminopyrine or sulpyrine as an active ingredient and vitamins. In February and March 1965, deaths considered to be caused by ampoule cold remedies were reported in Chiba, Shizuoka and Osaka and other locations. In total, 38 people died for few years foregoing the time and attracted the attention of the media. Eventually, MHW directed the pharmaceutical manufacturers to voluntarily discontinue sales of the preparation.

4) SMON is the abbreviation of "subacute myelo-optico neuropathy." Chinoform, an intestinal drug, is considered to be causally related to SMON. Patients have severe disturbance of perception/pain in lower extremities after having gastrointestinal disorders such as diarrhea/abdominal pain. Since around 1955 or so, neurological inflammation and paralysis of lower bodies of unknown cause were reported from patients treated for gastrointestinal diseases and considered to be rare neurological disorders in early days. SMON was recognized as a drug disaster when Prof. Tadao Tsubaki, Nigata University released the research result suggesting the relation between SMON and chinoform in 1970.

5) Chloroquine was developed for the treatment of malaria in Germany. It was introduced to the Japanese market in 1955 and was approved supplementally for the indications of chronic nephritis, nephropathy of pregnancy, chronic rheumatoid arthritis, systemic erythematodes and other diseases one after another. In 1959, chloroquine-induced retinopathy with main symptom of defect of visual field caused by impairment of fundus macula and narrowing of retinal blood vessels as an ADR to chloroquine was first reported abroad, and the number of cases of chloroquine-

induced retinopathy increased gradually since 1962. The drug disaster spread because MHW knew about chloroquine-induced retinopathy but did not supply the information to the public immediately and directed discontinuation of manufacturing but not recall.

6) A tragic fatal event caused by drug interaction took place in patients treated concurrently with sorivudine, a herpes zoster treatment drug, and fluorouracil anticancer drug. In the package insert, the risk of concurrent use of the drugs was mentioned but pharmaceutical companies failed to sufficiently supply the information to healthcare professionals. It was pointed out that the awareness of healthcare professionals, i.e. prescribing doctors and dispensing pharmacists, was also low.

Exercises

1. つぎの 1 ～ 34 の語に対応する英単語または英熟語を本文から選び出して書き込み，また発音しなさい（動詞は原形を記入しなさい）。

	Japanese	English		Japanese	English
1	医薬品		9	排泄	
2	最高の		10	時期尚早の,早すぎる	
3	健康増進		11	基準	
4	正当性		12	上にあげる	
5	安全性		13	合理化する,能率化する	
6	吸収		14	修復,改造	
7	分布		15	新薬	
8	代謝		16	予想,予測	

28 Unit A Pharmaceutical Science

	Japanese	English		Japanese	English
17	市場性, 商品価値		26	急性毒性	
18	収益性		27	亜急性毒性	
19	臨床的		28	慢性毒性	
20	見込みのある		29	暫定的に	
21	特許出願		30	副作用	
22	知的財産		31	ペニシリン・ショック	
23	分析化学		32	サリドマイド	
24	品質管理		33	抗生物質	
25	動物実験		34	感染症	

  2. つぎの各文が本文の内容と一致するものにはT(True), 一致しないものにはF(False)を, 文末の(   )に記入しなさい。

 (1) Recently, the drug development period before the use by general patients, has been reduced to about 5 years by the effort made by companies who demand acceleration of the R&D speed and patients who want to use new drugs. (   )

 (2) Japan, the U.S. and Europe are all concerned with escalating medical expenses. In particular, in Japan falling of birth rate and aging of population are remarkable. (   )

 (3) The process of drug development is roughly divided into planning stage and development stage. (   )

 (4) The development stage is divided into non-clinical studies performed using animals and clinical studies. (   )

 (5) Clinical studies performed for the first time in humans are called Phase III studies and are performed with strict caution under restricted conditions. (   )

 (6) The modern history of drugs is the history of drug disaster. No drug is free from ADRs. (　　)

3. つぎの日本語の各文を（　　）の中の語を用いて英語の文にしなさい（必要があれば単語を適切な形に変換しなさい）。

（1）現代人の生活は，化学物質によって大いに改善されてきた。例を挙げてみると，医薬品，化粧品，食品添加物，家庭用品，工業化学製品，建築資材など多くのものが，化学物質として世に見出され利用されてきた。(improve, utensil)

（2）インフルエンザと普通の風邪は，原因となるウイルスが違う。インフルエンザはインフルエンザウイルスによって，普通の風邪はアデノウイルス，ライノウイルス，細菌などが原因で起こる。(cause, adenovirus, rhinovirus)

（3）ジェネリック医薬品は，新薬に比べて大幅な開発コスト削減と開発期間の短縮が可能なため，新薬と同じ成分・同じ効き目でありながら，その価格は平均すると新薬の約半額に抑えられる。そのため患者の薬代の負担を軽減するだけでなく，国全体の医療費節減にも大きく貢献することができる。(suppress, It contributes to medical-expenses reduction.)

Unit A　Pharmaceutical Science

（4）現在，入院患者の少なくとも30％は抗生物質による治療を一つ，もしくはそれ以上受けており，生死に関わる何百万種もの感染症が治療されている。(inpatient, treat)

（5）日本人の生活が豊かになり，公衆衛生の向上，医学の進歩および保健・医療の充実とともに，赤痢，コレラ，結核などの伝染病は，治療法が確立され不治の病ではなくなった。しかし，治療が難しく，慢性の経過をたどる疾病もいまだ存在し，このような疾病を難病とよんでいる。(establish, intractable disease, chronic progress)

4. つぎの各問いに英語で答えなさい。

（1）May an antibiotic cure any kinds of disease?

（2）What will the chemical substance, not being a new drug which multiplied vast cost and time for a research and development, be reproduced in?

Chapter 2 Why Does Drug Development Require Time and Money?

(3) What kind of fever pain-killer is that cold medicine of ampoule occurred successively the death accidents in Chiba, Shizuoka and Osaka in 1959?

(4) Why will be appeared again that needs to check the fact as there are side effects in the medicines which has been used conventionally for many years?

(5) What kind of case must a patient care about in daily when a patient takes different medicines, although the death by drugs interaction have occurred frequently?

(6) May the development of the science and technology be regarded that the life of people will be rich and the world peace is promoted really?

Chapter 3 Are the Plant Materials as Both Medicines and Cosmetics Sufficient for?

3.1 Present Status and World Activity about Medicinal Plants Originated for the Drug

In the world of biology, people break out the change of consciousness to the natural resources in the 21st century, and have been approached to the new correspondence in the nation level to the profit distribution with the foreign country through Convention on Biological Diversity (CBD). The biggest worth of biological diversity shows ecological worth, and the conservation of biological diversity overlaps with nature conservation exactly. The one that I lost is not able to return it to the source. The biological diversity is also the guideline to healthy the earth environment including a human being. However, the real worth to the biological diversity through CBD is not acknowledged in the developing countries.

3.2 The United States has Not Yet Ratified the CBD. Why has Not United State Ratified it to this Treaty?

One possible explanation for this delay relates to the initiation of a large biodiversity project by a major U.S. pharmaceutical company in collaboration with a Costa Rican research institute. In a joint public, corporate and academic enterprise known around the world as the 'INBio-Merck Costa Rica System', this project has successfully negotiated the exclusive rights to research and develop the biological resources of a region of Costa Rica. The name INBio is an abbreviation of Instituto Nacional de Biodiversidad (Costa Rica Biological Diversity Research Institute), a private, nonprofit institute that has operated as a national organization since its inception by presidential decree in

1989. In addition to research for the utilization and conservation of biodiversity, the key objectives of this institute are encapsulated in activities towards the production of a national inventory of biological resources (incorporating the collation of biological collections in herbaria and museums, and the production of checklists and distribution maps for all species of plants and animals) and the appropriate management of the data involved. Furthermore, the institute represents a global model for the enrichment of research capacity through, for example, the training of personnel in taxonomy, as well as in the development of biological resources through bioprospecting under contractual cooperation with overseas pharmaceutical companies. More recently, INBio has also established an academic park next to its headquarters, signaling a shift towards environmental education.

3.3 The INBio-Merck Costa Rica System is Presently Suspended Following Termination of the Contract

With respect to its stance on the utilization of plant genetic resources, the United States therefore appears to be pursuing a program in which collaborative development has been prioritised; whilst this should not entail the indiscriminate use of biodiversity, is it evident that the U.S. considers free access to resources as essential? Research and development under the INBio-Merck Costa Rica System is presently suspended due to cessation of the contract.

During a five-year secondment to a medicinal plant research project organized by the National Wet Tropical Natural Resource Research Center under the auspices of the Amazon Agricultural Research Cooperation Plan in Brazil, the present author once had the opportunity to visit the New York Botanical Garden in the Bronx suburb of New York. The visit had been arranged in order to facilitate identification of plant specimens from South America, and drew on the expertise of Dr. Douglas, a plant taxonomist specializing in the higher plants of the Amazon region of eastern Brazil and the Guiana highland, and Dr. Henrique, then senior curator of Central American Botany. Though unable to examine all relevant collections because construction work for the renovation of the large greenhouse and development of the new Annex Specimen Gallery was underway, it was a truly eye-opening experience to find the specimens impeccably arranged and curated as if living fossils, each with detailed label notes recording the precise collection locality. This conscientiousness gave the impression that U.S. researchers had been anticipating the present era of plant resource nationalism for some time — and that an internationally binding treaty, if not the CBD, would one day be enforced. Without knowing the exact level of investment, it was at least apparent that significant sums of money had been allocated from the national budget for the construction and maintenance of the herbarium, and that this interest has, for the past two centuries, sustained the meticulous recording of data pertaining to much of the planet's endangered botanical heritage. It was clear that the U.S.'s approach to resource management fundamentally differed from that of Japan.

In general, the potential of plant resources in developing countries remains poorly understood. Furthermore, the effective utilization of plant resources — a key objective of the CBD — has not been realized due to the substantial costs involved in the commercialization of new drugs derived from plants. In view of this situation, this article argues that the surest way of ensuring the conservation of the natural environment whilst delivering sustainable development, is for methods for the sustainable and effective utilization of plant resources to be developed by economically stable countries, such as Japan, with part of the profits derived through subsequent commercialization being returned to ameliorate livelihoods in the less-developed areas from which the plants were sourced.

It is asserted here that the single most significant theme of the 21st Century is harmony between humans and nature — this harmony is essential for the development of a truly prosperous society. We must resolve cross-boundary environmental issues by recognizing our responsibility for handing over this resource-rich planet to future generations.

3.4 What is the Medicine Produced from the Plant? In Case of *Taxus baccata* as Western Yew

The alkaloid taxol was first successfully isolated from yew, *Taxus brevifolia* Hort. ex Gord. (a member of the Taxaceae family that grows wild in the mountains of Oregon State in USA) in 1971. It drew widespread interest throughout the scientific community when its carcinostatic properties were first realized in pre-clinical trials, and strong anti-tumor activity was recognized in subsequent test at the U.S. National Cancer Institute (NCI). It also was found to be effective against various cancerous cells where cisplatin, another carcinostatic substance, showed no suppressive action, and is currently available on the market.

Moreover, the same Genus as yew tree, the instantaneous effect over hay fever or articular rheumatism rheumatoid arthritis is expected as examples of application other than cancer, and the related product has also come to be sold to the "Yunnan yew tree" as *Taxus yunnanensis* while research progress.

As drugs, the vaccination which various antibiotics which begin penicillin in ancient times and a microbe makes, and an animal were made to make is mentioned. Moreover, although use of gene modification technology in recent years has typical production of a human insulin biotechnology, such as an elucidation of a sick mechanism, an evaluation test of a sample, and fabrication of a sick model animal, is highly used in various scenes, and many antibiotics, an tumor drug, hormone, an antibody, and various diagnostic products are made from the medical field by the microbe and the animal cell.

It seems that gene synthesis examination of man finishes and arrival of the genome omnipotence age came now. Illness and a constitution are also beginning to understand a closely related gene because genomics progressed and the analysis of the information for every individual and every illness and accumulation also progressed. In the future, it will become possible to also fully perform gene diagnosis and gene therapy. Moreover, the medical-supplies medication which is suited the individual constitution and which is effective and has side effects is considered that what is called medical treatment tailored to individual patients also progresses. The artificial organ transplant which will have neither regeneration medicine nor rejection in various organizations and internal organs from now on will be attained using the technology of an organization and internal-organs cultivation. I want to imagine the future which can detect many illnesses easily on an early stage by progress of advanced and quick a diagnostic product and inspection.

3.5 What is the Medicine Produced from the Plant?
In Case of *Camptotheca acuminata* as Happy Tree

Camptothecine is another carcinostatic alkaloid that, like taxol, was first discovered by researchers at the NCI. Though first isolated from the Chinese plant *Camptotheca acuminata* Decne (Nyssaceae), its occurrence also in *Nothapodytes nimmonianus*, syn. *Nothapodytes foetida* (Icacinaceae) and *Merrilliodendron megacarpum* (Hemsl.)

Sleum. (both Icacinaceae), *Ervatamia heyneana* Cooke (Apocynaceae), and *Ophiorrhiza mungos* Bartl. ex DC. (Rubiaceae) has since been confirmed. Camptothecine was developed by a Japanese pharmaceutical company, and a derivative, irinotecan, came onto the market as the first anticancer drug in Japan under the generic name Campto. Several other anti-cancer compounds are derived from plants, including vincristine and vinblastine, both isolated from *Catharanthus roseus* G. Don (Apocynaceae). Other similar indole-alkaloids are also known to exist in the Apocynaceae. Vincristine and vinblastine have strong anti-tumor activity and have been approved as medicines to cure leukemia. The number of medical specialists who attempt a treatment mixture consisting of a plant-derived carcinostatic compound and steroid (such as the R-CHOP method which is used against B-cell malignant lymphatic tumors) has recently increased. However, this approach also requires chemical treatment methods that are not yet permitted in Japan, and they are commonly not covered by national health insurance.

Many new plant-derived drugs such as these surely still await discovery, especially in developing countries where most of the Earth's plant resources are concentrated. However, developing nations increasingly adopt a competitive stance with regard to bio-prospecting, and continue to tighten regulations pertaining to plant inventory and ethno-botanical research. This is exacerbated by fears that drugs effective in the treatment of disease may become scarce in the future. Meanwhile, the destruction of natural areas alongside rapidly global economic development stands to destroy many potential plant sources of future medicines, and the traditional use of plants as medicines by indigenous populations is diminishing as exchanges between populations become more pronounced (Imanishi & Nihonyanagi, 1997). This is particularly remarkable in societies of small minority populations, where oral exchanges of knowledge pertaining to plants are decreasing even before the disappearance of their familiar forests, and well before ethno-botanical studies and written records are made.

Collaborative research focusing on plants cultivated in medicinal plant collections can make a vital contribution to the conservation and sustainable utilization of the natural environment through the technologies and experiences that have been accumulated in botanical gardens and related institutes in Japan. In this respect, I believe that the public at large increasingly recognizes the profound significance of medicinal plant gardens.

3.6 Positioning of Plant Biotechnology, and Production of the Medicinal Substance by Biotechnology

It will be classified into animal cell cultivation system biotechnology, microbe system biotechnology, and plant system biotechnology as biotechnology is divided roughly. Although animal cell cultivation system biotechnology is in use about the manufacture fields, such as medicines, at present, risks what does not have fear of disease germ infection, such as mad cow disease, in the animal cell to be used must be used, are high. Moreover, in order to obtain the serum to be used, the subject seen from the ethical sides, such as animal protection, is posing a problem in Europe and America.

Since it differs from an animal or higher forms of life like a plant in microbe system biotechnology, while there is an advantage, such as there being comparatively few technical issues which should be conquered and excelling. The great expectation as useful substance manufacture processes, such as medicines what a substance producible as medical-supplies manufacture technology used for humans etc., is limited as substance without sugar chain ornamentation. That has a field which is hard to carry out.

Chapter 3 Are the Plant Materials as Both Medicines and Cosmetics Sufficient for?

On the other hand, since the growth speed of plant system biotechnology is slow, although substance production takes time to it, it becomes possible for producing the plant of the same character in large quantities through seeds, and becomes possible for producing a useful substance stably.

Conventionally, if it is not an animal, possibility of being producible, such as medical supplies considered to be impossible, will be found out, and it is thought possible by developing this method to replace the conventional medical-supplies manufacture process. It leads to the ability to contribute to global warming prevention, such as CO_2 fixed O_2 discharge by the photosynthesis which is the vegetable big feature when this method spreads, and also is expected as environmental harmony type manufacture technology of having a possibility that it can contribute to absorption purification of the toxic substance

Table 3.1 Comparison of production system by an animal / a microbe / plant biotechnology

Characteristics	Animal (cell cultivation)	Microorganism	Plants
proliferation rate	rapid	very rapid	slow
production cost	expensive	cheap	very cheap
carbon dioxide mineralization energy consumption	exhausting yes	exhausting yes	absorption fixation
restoration & storage	freezing /cold	freezing /cold	room temperature
product safety management	essential such as BSE	necessary	no

動物・微生物・植物バイオ技術による生産系比較
特に，植物バイオテクノロジーを活用した医薬品などの物質生産プロセスを考えた場合，植物栽培系が環境負荷の少ない環境調和型プロセスであること，生産設備などへの投資やランニングコストが従来の 1/1,000 程度で製造できる見込みがあること，および，動物細胞に感染する病原菌に対する安全性といったことが大きな利点となっている。

in soil etc. Moreover, producing the herbal medicine ingredient which is made to contain an ingredient effective in the plant as foods for health maintenance and prevention of a disease and by which production is made difficult except the vegetable system etc. also expects the application deployment which can be carried out only in vegetable system biotechnology (**Table 3.1, Table 3.2**).

Table 3.2 Examples such as useful protein produced with a plant

pharmaceutical product	antibody	human herpesvirus antibody
	vaccine	虫歯菌 / hepatitis type B virus / cholera vibrio / *Escherichia coli* / 豚下痢症ウイルス
	enzyme	anticoagulant enzyme / antibacterial enzyme / digestive enzyme
	blood products	albumin / hemoglobin / blood coagulation factor
	immunity fortifier	interferon, interleukin 10
	others	sterol / squalene
chemical products	Industrial use enzyme	cellulase / amylase / キシラナーゼ
	Biological decomposition plastic / polyester	

植物で生産された有用蛋白質などの例
米国を筆頭に欧州やアジア諸国などの国々は，世界のリーダーシップをとるため先を競って研究開発を進めており，研究開発対象はワクチン，抗体，蛋白製剤などの蛋白性医薬品が圧倒的に多く，産業用酵素や化粧品・健康食品原料，油脂などについても研究が進められている。

3.7 Industrialization Project that Prevents the Disappearing of Plant Material for Cosmetics

Since 2002, the Toyota Motor Corporation's environmental activity support program has funded development work in Lo-Monthang the capital city of the Kingdom of Mustang in western Nepal. The foci of this work have been the construction of a museum of herbal medicine as an annex to the Lo-Monthang Traditional Medicine and Astrology School (a training centre for young doctors from Tibet), and the development of a highland medicinal herb farm. The work has fused environmental objectives with those that promote development, with the overall aim of ameliorating the quality of life locally.

3.7.1 Project background

(1) **Funding**　　Funding is administered via Toyota's Global 500 Project, which was initiated in 1999 as part of the United Nations Environment Program (UNEP). The Project offers financial support for NGOs to conduct environmental activities that aspire to deliver social, as well as environmental benefits, including environmental conservation and improvements for sustainable development. Since operations typically necessitate management of plant resources (incorporating wild plant species as well as those in use or known to be of some economic application), the Project is implemented according to the CBD. Its three primary objectives are: (i) the conservation of biological diversity, (ii) the sustainable use of the components of biological diversity, and (iii) the fair and equitable distribution of profits derived from utilization (i.e. benefit-sharing).

(2) **Local considerations**　　Lo-Monthang stands at 3,800 m above sea level in the Nepal Himalaya, and its name translates literally as "southern Tibet" (*Lo*) and "prayers for herbs in the fields where many herbs grow" (*Monthang*) (**Figures 3.1〜3.4**). It is located 80 km from Jomson (itself a 40 minute flight from Pokhara, Nepal's second largest city), a journey that can take four or five days on foot or by horse due to the steep topography and the absence of surfaced roads. Though it is situated at approximately the same latitude as Amami-Oshima in southern Japan, Lo-Monthang experiences a very dry climate and is exposed to strong winds. It is an area that has been

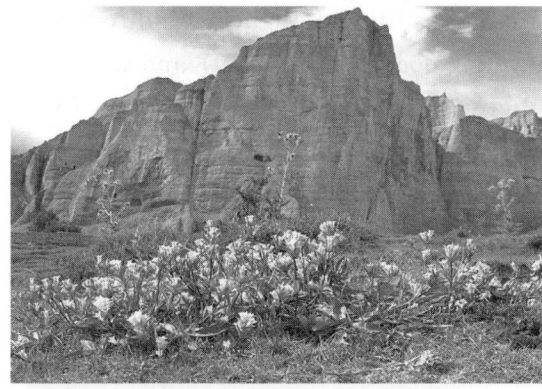

Figure 3.1 High-land of the kingdom of Lo-Monthang which meaning by the Pray Field of Medicinal Herbs on the South of Tibet

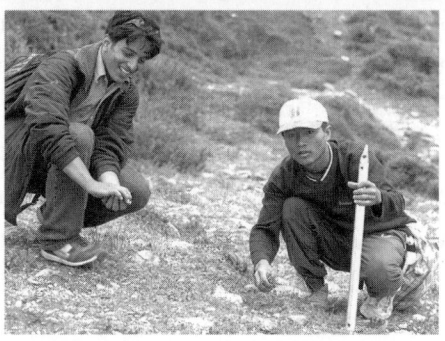

Figure 3.2 Experimental Station of Himalayan Herb Center-Lo upper Mustang, working with Amchi's (Tibetan Medical Doctor's) Stuffs

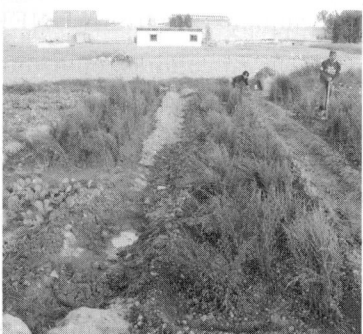

Figure 3.3 Cultivating some medicinal herbs having value of income in Experimental Station of Himalayan Herb Center-Lo upper Mustang

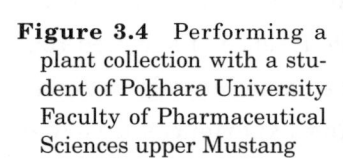

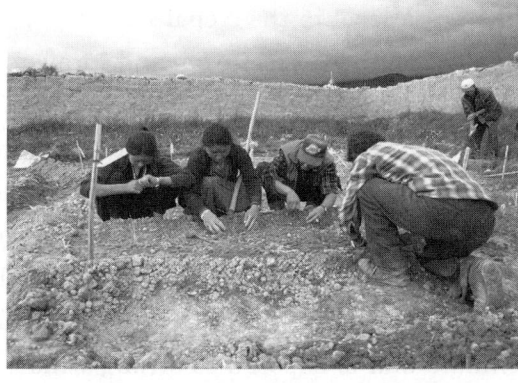

Figure 3.4 Performing a plant collection with a student of Pokhara University Faculty of Pharmaceutical Sciences upper Mustang

strongly influenced by Tibetan culture: Tibetan Buddhism is deeply rooted in the local population, and indigenous forms of medicine draw predominantly on Tibetan techniques. In addition, the area has long relied on trade with India and Tibet because local agricultural yields are insufficient. More recently, however, new roads have been built from the Chinese side, leading to a reduction in reliance on yaks for trade, and a demographic shift in young people from rural areas to urban centers (such as Katmandu) in search of work.

3.7.2 Lo-Monthang Herbal Medicine Museum

Permission to build a museum of herbal medicine in Lo-Monthang was granted by Amchi Gyatso Bista, a traditional doctor at the Lo-Kunphen Men-Tsee Khang Traditional Herbal Medicine Clinic and School. Building materials were transported to the site by the end of 2002. Amchi Gyatso Bista visited Japan in early spring in 2003, to receive training and to discuss the design of the museum with staff in Japan. A meeting was also held at the Kochi Prefectural Makino Botanical Garden where progress was discussed with the garden's director and project collaborator, Prof. Dr. Tetsuo Koyama. Support was also received from Japanese Cue letter, a member of the exhibition design staff at the Makino Botanical Garden. Final plans for the museum were completed after two weeks of consultation and review.

Construction of the first floor was completed by early September 2003 with the local cooperation of Amchi Tenzin Bista, Amchi Gyatso's younger brother, and his students. Construction was recommenced in May of the following year, and presently construction of the second floor and the interior is nearing completion. Equipment and facilities (including display cases, work stands to prepare samples, bookcases for technical books, a staff conference room, and a museum shop) will be installed by the end of 2007.

3.7.3 Lo-Monthang highland medicinal herb farm for crop trials and education

This project was started in March 2002 to facilitate self-sufficient cultivation and systematic preservation of plant material for the local preparation of herbal medicines under the direction of Tenzin Bista, director of the Lo-Kunphen Men-Tsee Khang medicinal herb farm. Project development here has been challenging but, after four years, the farm has been greatly improved and medical students are now taught methods for cultivating medicinal plants to be used in daily medical care.

In this project, about the high medicinal herb and cosmetics materials plant of added value which were found out by joint research with a university. In cooperation with a Japanese company or a local NGO organization, commission cultivation with LOC (local organization committee) is promoted so that it can use also as a general-purpose homemade agent to the Tibet doctor. Furthermore, the policy for which it does not depend on exploitation from nature by guiding cultivation techniques by dispatch of a specialist has been devised.

Moreover, it is also another purpose to establish the way of cash earnings in the farmer who advances plant industrialization from the effect-of-a-medicine activity ingredient obtained from strange plant resources, and belongs to LOC in accordance with the contents a contract of was made with NGO as a practical farmer. This project is started and five years are about to pass. It is visible as if the desirable situation of entrusting and purchasing cultivation of a materials plant is also produced and a cosmetics company began to get off the ground at last, but there is no change in the situation where it does not escape from mind still more.

Preparing the government initiative type resource agreement which strengthened protection of plant resources and ownership must avoid. A threshold is only made high to the company which enters into the plant industrial field, and superfluous expectation also serves as hindrance of development, and a company is sometimes often withdrawn from this field. If industrialization does not progress, the way of the cash earnings of a spot will be shut. Finally, are there really any enough materials of the medicine using a plant or cosmetics? Thinking that its medicinal demand also increases in population on the earth although it is hard to say the answer at a word seems to be very natural resources. In the modern society where the demand of precious natural resources and the balance of supply are collapsing, it is also a fact that the voice which thinks the protection of nature and an environmental problem as important is increasing. We also know the value of anxiety nature for exhaustion of plant resources. And production of the medicines and cosmetics materials which made full use of biotechnology in order to keep loss of the plant resources about which researchers are helped by many supporters, and we are anxious daily to decrease plant resources, and for protecting these resources the research on establishment and the plant propagation of plant cultivation techniques will surely be continued constantly.

The plant research on establishment about the production of medicines and cosmetics materials using biotechnology, and both vegetative propagation and cultivation techniques will surely be continued constantly. I believe that the harmony between nature and human activities is essential to develop a truly prosperous society in the 21st century. We must resolve environmental issues that cross national borders by recognizing our responsibility for handing over this resource-rich planet to the next generation.

46   Unit A   Pharmaceutical Science

Exercises

1. つぎの 1～19 の語に対応する英単語または英熟語を本文から選び出して書き込み，また発音しなさい（動詞は原形を記入しなさい）。

	Japanese	English		Japanese	English
1	利益配分		11	拒絶反応	
2	生物多様性条約		12	植物バイオテクノロジー	
3	生態学的		13	動物愛護	
4	ナショナル・インベントリー		14	ワクチン	
5	高等植物		15	血液製剤	
6	持続可能な発展		16	免疫増強剤	
7	米国がん研究所		17	生分解プラスチック	
8	関節リウマチ		18	産業用酵素	
9	抗体		19	拒絶反応	
10	人工臓器				

2. つぎの各文が本文の内容と一致するものには T(True)，一致しないものには F(False) を，文末の（   ）に記入しなさい。

（1）生物多様性条約を通じて他国との利益配分に対する国家レベルでの新たな対応に迫られてきたが，その真の価値は途上国にはあまり認知されていない。（   ）

（2）21世紀が真に豊かな社会として持続的に発展していくためには，環境と人間の活動との調和のことより，環境悪化の防止策をすぐにでも策定するほうが重要である。（   ）

（3）地球上で大半の植物資源を有する途上国側では民族植物学研究などの資源調査に対する規制を強化する一つの理由として，彼らの固有の

植物文化を守ることが挙げられる。（　　）

（4）地球上には，3万〜5万種の高等植物が知られている。（　　）

（5）アルカロイド成分のカンプトテシンの誘導体であるイリノテカンは，日本初の植物由来の制がん剤である。（　　）

（6）植物産業分野の現地参入が，開発途上国への経済支援に影響を大きく及ぼし，直接現金収入の道を開く。（　　）

3． つぎの日本語の各文を（　　）の中の語を用いて英語の文にしなさい（必要があれば単語を適切な形に変換しなさい）。

（1）米国は植物遺伝資源をむやみに取り扱うのではなく，目的に沿って利用する方法を優先し，資源の自由なアクセスが十分に確保されなければならないと考えた。（thought）

（2）バイオテクノロジーを大別すると動物細胞培養系バイオ，微生物系バイオおよび植物系バイオに分類される。主流の動物細胞培養系バイオは，近年狂牛病などの病原菌感染のリスクや動物を利用した血清生産が動物愛護などの倫理的側面から問題視されている。（divide, cell culture system）

（3）植物バイオテクノロジーを活用した医薬品などの物質生産プロセスは，環境負荷の少ない環境調和型プロセスであり，生産設備などへの投資やランニングコストを低く抑えられるといった利点が多い。（advantage, utilize）

（4）ヒマラヤ山岳地域において，一見相反するように見えるが環境を保全する事業と産業化を振興する事業を同時に行うことで，より環境に配慮した現地立脚型のモデル事業を展開してきた。(consider, industrialization)

（5）植物資源の枯渇を憂い自然の尊さを知っている研究者らは，植物資源の損失を防ぐためにバイオテクノロジーによる植物の無菌増殖研究に取り組んでいる。しかし，その成果を発揮するまでには，さらに多くの時間と費用を要する。(exhaustion, tackle)

4．つぎの各問いに英語で答えなさい。
（1）Will a poppy substitute cultivation project for drug destruction improve local poverty, and it really promote world peace?

Chapter 3 Are the Plant Materials as Both Medicines and Cosmetics Sufficient for?

(2) Are raw materials of medicine enough?

(3) How do the present conditions of biological diversity become?

(4) What kind of medical supplies from plant origin is there?

(5) What is a name of plant originated from China containing camptothecine as the production raw materials of anticancer agent irinotecan?

(6) Why do we have to avoid resources agreement of government-led model which strengthened plant resources and protection of proprietary rights?

Unit B　Infectious Diseases

Chapter 4　Zoonosis

Some pathogens and pests can infect commonly to human-beings and animals, and consequently infected animals could transmit diseases to human. They are called zoonosis.

　Typical examples would be rabies, toxocarosis (*Toxocara canis* and *Toxocara cati*) and toxoplasmosis. Rabies is a viral zoonotic disease that causes acute encephalitis (inflammation of the brain) in mammals. The infection could reach death unless prompt subsequent vaccinations to be made after bitten-injury from infected animals such as dogs, cats and wild animals like rabbits and raccoons. Toxocarosis could cause both eye and gut infections. The medication method is different from the ways for animals, so that consultation with specialized doctors is essential and it is wise not to ask veterinarians. Toxosoplasmosis is caused by *Toxoplasma gondii* that is common protozoa to avians and mammalians including human. Generally speaking, it is inapparent infection and there is no major concern, however, when the embryo is infected, it could cause abortion of the fetus or **substantial** damage to the baby.

　Q (Query) fever is caused by a bacterium species, **Coxiella burnetii** which is a relative of **Rickettsia** and **Legionella**. The bacterium species can be born by mites and also the dairy products such

Notes :
Toxocara canis and *Toxocara cati*「原虫の仲間」, veterinarian「獣医」
Toxoplasma gondii「原虫の仲間」, *Coxiella burnetii, Rickettsia, Legionella*「細菌類の仲間」

as natural milk and environments like soil and air at the infested livestock houses. Unfortunately, the concrete prevention system is not established, but it can be cured with proper treatment including antibiotics administration.

Athlete foot can be shared among human and animals as dermatophytosis is also regarded as causes for zoonosis. Echinococcosis is endemic in Hokkaido, and it is caused by **Echinocuccus**. This is vectored mainly by wild rats and their predator, foxes, but it is very serious sickness as to cause liver mal-function.

Global communities concern the outbreaks of various types of infectious diseases in the past decades. Many of them are known to be mediated by various animals.

Suspicion was made to mammalians such as masked palm civet cats (ハクビシン , *Paguma larvata*, **Figure 4.1**(a)) and raccoons when SARS (Severe Acute Respiratory Syndrome) outbroke in Asia and indeed those mammalians could carry the pathogens. Now it is known that SARS corona virus is hosted in nature by a bat species *Rhinolophus sinicus*.

Ebola virus, was found fist at Zaire and Sudan in 1976, which causes the devastating disease with fever and hemorrhage, reaching a very high death rate in a short period. It was reported that Fruit bats (Figure 4.1(b)) is the natural host of the ebola virus (Nature 438: p.575, (2003)). It was suggested that the public enlightenment of the prohibition of hunting wild creatures and the reduction on the exposure to the host species, as the local people in the ebola endemic areas, often eat the fruit bats.

Notes :
Echinocuccus「原虫の仲間」, *Rhinolophus sinicus*「キクガシラコウモリ」
Fruit bats「オオコウモリ」

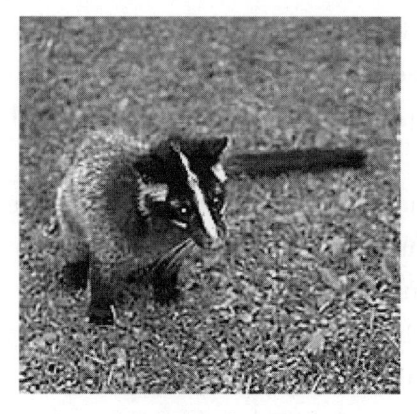

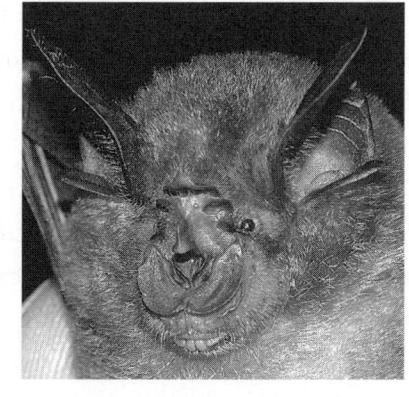

(a) Masked Palm Civet Cat
(*Paguma larvata*)

(b) Chinese Rufous Horseshoe Bat
(*Rhinolophus sinicus*)

Figure 4.1 Which animal is the suspect carrying SARS?
(http://www.bio.bris.ac.uk/research/bats/China%20bats/rhinophus sinicus.htm, http://beta.uniprot.org/taxonomy/9675)

Marburg haemorrhagic fever is also caused by biological agent, a single strand RNA virus, which was reported by the incidences happened at Marburg and Frankfurt, Germany and Beograde at Yugoslavia in 1967, which made seven people died out of the 31 victims. It was first attributed to monkeys imported from Uganda, but later on the epidemiological and animal studies, also attributed to a fruit bat species.

Also species-specific pathogens such as viruses, could alter its host-specificity by making gradual evolution by their exposure to the human. A good example would be avaian influenza virus. It could be attributed to the emerging demands and consumption of domestic avians such as chicken and the eggs. Poultry industry in Asia, was not well controlled to the exposure to the wild host birds such as common ducks, the wild birds'excrement contaminated at narrow and filthy chicken ranches. Also commercial trade is commonly made with live poultry, so that there are increased possibilities to human inhale the viral agents via excrements from the live birds.

Human pathogenic agent might have been infected to animals. Proteinaceous infectious particle (prion) causes the disease, Creutzfeldt-Jakob disease (CJD) in human by making involuntary movements and rapid progress in dementia. BSE's (bovine spongiform encephalopathy, 狂牛病) origin might be to CJD, not vice versa. (The origin of bovine spongiform encephalopathy: the human prion disease hypothesis. Lancet 366: pp.856 〜 861, (2005)).

It cannot be denied on globalization and the international movement of human-beings day-to-day basis. However, there shall be alleviating the issues by considering some elements: knowledge and education on hygiene and sanitation, recognition of the change of the value of own life, ethics and legal regulation in trade and transport of animals. Thus, it may be reconsidered to settle down the borderlines for interactions of wild creatures and human lives with relevant public educational elements.

Exercises

1. つぎの 1 〜 46 の語に対応する英単語または英熟語を本文から選び出して書き込み，また発音しなさい（動詞は原形を記入しなさい）。

	Japanese	English		Japanese	English
1	病原		6	傷害	
2	害虫		7	内臓	
3	感染する		8	肝臓	
4	人獣共通感染症		9	獣医	
5	咬む		10	狂犬病	

Note:

Creutzfeldt-Jakob disease (CJD)「クロイツフェルト-ヤコブ病」

Unit B　Infectious Diseases

	Japanese	English		Japanese	English
11	犬・猫回虫症		29	媒介する	
12	トキソプラズマ症		30	仲介する	
13	急性		31	生物を捕えて食う	
14	脳炎		32	汚染する	
15	炎症		33	予防	
16	脳		34	発生する	
17	ほ乳類		35	宿主（となる）	
18	鳥類		36	出血性の	
19	不顕性感染		37	疫学的	
20	原虫		38	（罹病）発生	
21	胎児(受胎後3カ月以内)		39	特異性	
22	胎児		40	家禽業	
23	流産		41	排泄物	
24	水虫		42	吸引する	
25	皮膚糸状菌症		43	不随意の	
26	風土性		44	衛生学	
27	エキノコックス症		45	公衆衛生	
28	包虫		46	生き物	

　2．つぎの各文が本文の内容と一致するものにはT(True)，一致しないものにはF(False)を，文末の（　　）に記入しなさい．
　(1) Human pathogenic agent might have been infected to animals. (　)

(2) Viral agents cannot be inhaled by human. (　)
(3) Ebola virus does not cause a serious disease. (　)
(4) Typical examples of zoonosis are toxocarosis and toxosoplasmosis. (　)
(5) Q (Query) fever cannot be cured with medication such by administration of antibiotics. (　)

3．つぎの日本語の各文を（　）の中の語を用いて英語の文にしなさい（必要があれば単語を適切な形に変換しなさい）。
(1) 水虫は，皮膚糸状菌症の一種であり，人と動物の間で相互感染する人畜共通感染症である。(infect, mutual, dermatophytosis, zoonosis)

(2) 多様な感染症の発生は，過去数十年の間に世界的な問題事項となってきている。(outbreak, decade, global)

(3) SARSはハクビシンや狸が宿主で広がったわけではない。コウモリの類いが天然の宿主であると考えられている。(host, spread, masked palm civet cat, regard)

(4) マールブルグウイルスは出血熱を生じ，感染者の死亡率は高い。このウイルスもコウモリが宿主でこの類いによって媒介される。(haemorrhagic fever, mediate, cause)

56　Unit B　Infectious Diseases

（5）トキソプラズマ症は，原虫によって引き起こされる。通常では，人では不顕性でことだった病状が現れるわけではない。しかし，妊婦では胎児への影響が高く，流産やかなりの障害が出産後の嬰児（えい）に現われることがある。(substantial, protozoa, abortion, influence)

4．つぎの各問いに英語で答えなさい。

（1）What is zoonosis?

（2）Why wild fruit bats should be avoided?

（3）What is the precaution when approaching to wild life?

（4）What is the prion?

（5）What is typical example of zoonosis?

Chapter 5 Hope for Incurable Infection Diseases and Prevention: Malaria

A bite from a mosquito infected with certain parasites may trigger malaria. Most malaria infections cause flu-like symptoms such as high fever, chills, muscle pain, and diarrhea, and these symptoms tend to come and go in cycles as the disease progresses. Recent analyses show that an estimated toll of 300–500 million new infections and 1.5–3 million deaths occurred annually.

The development of a malaria vaccine is a formidable challenge. Despite a relatively intense and systematic research effort conducted since the 1960s and clinical trials of a large number of candidate vaccine with a range of delivery systems designed to induce protective antibody or cell-mediated immune responses against the sporozoite in circulation, the infected hepatocyte or the parasitized erythrocyte, few humans have been protected. As compared to developing vaccines against viruses and bacteria, developing a vaccine against malaria is complicated by the complexity of the parasite as well as the complexity of the host's response to the parasite.

The feasibility of developing a malaria vaccine is suggested by two human models demonstrating that protective immunity can be induced by exposure to intact *Plasmodium falciparum* parasites. The first model is to design a vaccine which induces sterile immunity in humans by immunization with radiation-attenuated *P. falciparum* sporozoites to prevent all clinical manifestations of malaria. The second model is to design a vaccine which induces erythrocytic stage immunity to prevent death and severe disease of naturally acquired immunity. However, despite considerable efforts over the past decades, no vaccine candidate has proven sufficiently efficacious to warrant commercial development (**Figure 5.1**).

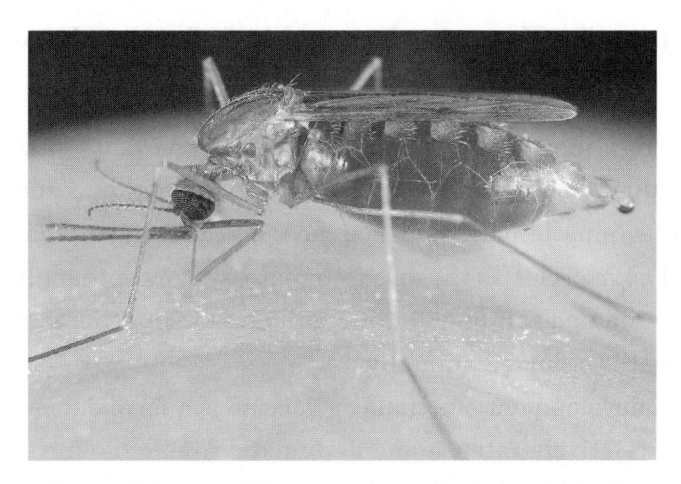

Figure 5.1 Anopheles mosquito vectoring malaria disease (http://www.cdc.gov/malaria/biology/mosquito/)

In 1996, an international consortium of genome scientists and funding agencies was formed to sequence the genome of *P. falciparum*. It was anticipated that the data deriving from related projects would facilitate the development of effective interventions against malaria, including vaccines, drugs and diagnostics. The genomic sequence of *P. falciparum* was completed and published in 2002, and additional erythorcite-surface-expressed parasite proteins have been identified. More recently, the gene expression profile during the different stages of the parasite life cycles has been completed. Putative hepatic-stage-specific proteins have also been identified through expressed sequence tag (EST) sequencing. In total, these data provide a set of bioinformatics corresponding to potential *P. falciparum* target antigens and evidence for expression of these genes in different stages of the parasite life cycle. This foundation can be exploited for the identification and prioritization of novel antigens and epitopes that may be targets of anti-malarial protective immunity.

Chapter 5 Hope for Incurable Infection Diseases and Prevention: Malaria

Exercises

1. つぎの1〜44の語に対応する英単語または英熟語を本文から選び出して書き込み，また発音しなさい（動詞は原形を記入しなさい）。

	Japanese	English		Japanese	English
1	寄生虫,寄生動物		21	寄生虫,寄生動物	
2	マラリア		22	実行可能性	
3	症候		23	マラリアの寄生虫	
4	寒け		24	殺菌した	
5	下痢		25	免疫性	
6	推測の,推定		26	予防注射,予防接種	
7	伝染体		27	放射	
8	毎年		28	弱力化した	
9	ワクチン		29	徴候	
10	手に負えない		30	有効な	
11	強烈な,集中的		31	認可する	
12	系統的,組織的な		32	協会,連合	
13	候補者		33	予期された	
14	胞子虫の種虫		34	促進する	
15	血液循環		35	介入	
16	肝細胞		36	診断学	
17	〜に寄生する		37	推定上の	
18	赤血球		38	発現配列タグ	
19	複雑な		39	生物情報学	
20	複雑さ		40	〜に対応する	

60　Unit B　Infectious Diseases

	Japanese	English		Japanese	English
41	活用された		43	優先順位	
42	識別，鑑定，検証		44	抗原決定基	

　2．つぎの各文が本文の内容と一致するものにはT(True)，一致しないものにはF(False)を，文末の（　）に記入しなさい。

　（1）Malaria is caused by a bite from a mosquito infected with certain parasite. (　)

　（2）The symptoms of malaria are high fever, chills, muscle pain, and diarrhea. (　)

　（3）Clinical trials of malaria vaccine have protected many humans from malaria successfully. (　)

　（4）Two models of developing malaria vaccine have been proven sufficiently effeicacious to warrant commercial development. (　)

　（5）Data base corresponding to potential infected malaria have been established recently. (　)

　3．つぎの日本語の各文を（　）の中の語を用いて英語の文にしなさい（必要があれば単語を適切な形に変換しなさい）。

　（1）最近の分析により，毎年約150～300万人がマラリアの感染で死んでしまう。(infect, malaria, annually)

　（2）1960年代以来かなりの研究努力を払ってきても，マラリアの感染から守られる人数は少ない。(effort, conduct, protect)

　（3）マラリアワクチンのデザインをする第一のモデルは，放射線照射で弱化した種虫を用いて人の体内の無菌免疫を誘導する方法である。(model, vaccine, induce, sterile immunity, radiation-attenuated sporozoite)

Chapter 5 Hope for Incurable Infection Diseases and Prevention: Malaria

（4）マラリアワクチンのデザインをする第二のモデルは，赤血球に入れる時期の免疫であり，自然獲得性疾病を予防する。(erythorocytic stage, naturally acquired immunity)

（5）ゲノム配列データは，強力なマラリアターゲット抗原に関与する一連の生物情報を提供する。(genomic, sequence, bioinformatics, correspond, potential, target, antigen)

4．つぎの各問いに英語で答えなさい。
（1）What may cause malaria infection?

（2）Why the developing a vaccine against malaria is more difficult than those of viruses and bacteria?

（3）How many models have been suggested to develop a malaria vaccine?

（4）What are the merits provided by the two models of developing a malaria vaccine?

（5）Who started the sequence of genome of malaria in 1996?

Unit C Genetic Disorders

Chapter 6 Dementious Disorders: Alzheimer's Disease

Dementious disorders have diversity such as cerebrovascular dementia(CD), Parkinson's disease (PD) and Alzheimer's disease (AD). This chapter focuses on AD, but short description is also made on CD and PD.

1. Cerebrovascular dementia (CD)

CD occurs commonly as one of senile dementious ailment. Symptom changes very suddenly from light patterns to serious conditions. The preventive efforts can be made by reducing the risks to vascular disorders such as atherosclerosis, hypertension, schemic heart disease, diabetics, hyperlipidemia. Thus, it is recommended to integrate a healthy diet, appropriate exercises and attention to daily behaviors in your life style.

2. Parkinson's disease (PD)

PD is a neuron system disorder which is associated with the shortage of the amount of dopamine in the brain and relative increase in the quantity of acetylcholine. PD associates with Lewy body syndrome which takes place by the degradation of the dopamine-driven neurons. The general appearance symptoms are: rigidity, resting tremor, postural instability, akinesia, and bradykinesia, and also often observation are seen such on the disorders in autonomic nervous system,

---

Notes :
Parkinson's disease「パーキンソン病」, Alzheimer's disease「アルツハイマー病」
dopamine「ドーパミン」, acetylcholine「アセチルコリン」
Lewy body syndrome「レビー小体症」

depression and dementia. The majority of the cases are independent occurrence based on individual neuro-physiological disorders, but minor portion of the patients have heritable events. Medicaments could help dealing with or slow-down the PD such as dopamine or nor-adrenalin associated materials. Some PD-related genes were reported recently, and endeavor is expected to make control of such genetic disorders and gene therapies.

3. Alzheimer's disease (AD)

AD associates with the cognitive impairments and the change of personality. The capacity could be decreased such by: defects of memory, disorientation, obstacles in learning, lack of attention and spatial sense, and ability reduction in resolving problems etc. and consequently overall social adaptability is decreased. AD progresses gradually and serious levels of AD could cause troubles in eating, changing cloths and communications, ending with no capacity living by oneself. There are two types on AD: 1) familial AD which is the minor portion of overall AD patients and the ailment controlled by locus at an autosomal chromosome with Mendelian inheritance, namely, it is a genetic disease and 2) senile dementia with Alzheimer's type (SDAT), which is the majority of the AD patients.

Pathological traits of AD are: brain tissue atrophy and appearance of the senile plaque in cerebral cortex. The senile plaque has the deposition of the beta-amyloid on cerebral cortex. Cerebral cortex is the gray-color layers of neurons which reside the surface of the cerebrum.

Could AD be avoided by daily efforts? There are epidemiological studies that eating more meats could increase the risk and alternatively the possibility of the occurrence of the AD could be reduced by having balanced diets with vegetables and fish.

The progress of the AD could be deterred by using medicaments.

Examples would be cholinesterase inhibitors such as donepezil hydrochloride or the comercial name is ARICEPT. The medicine could enhance the capacity of acetylcholine associated neurons, which lead to the recovery of the memory capacity.

Consideration: The patients with dementious disorders, especially with AD, would have persecution mania and/or hallucination with its disease progress. The stakeholders of the patients such as medical workers, social care-takers and family members should be sure that there are diversity of unusual and problematic behaviors such on abusive language, violence, unintentional loitering, and filthy conducts. But, patience and understanding with kind consideration, must be enhanced to care the patients that those who are very vulnerable. With the challenge in the modern medical sciences, sometimes the disorders can be associated with heritable genetic nature, and prejudice should not be made to the families or individuals with ancestral pedigree containing patients as discussed in Chapters 7 and 8.

Exercises

1．つぎの 1 ～ 46 の語に対応する英単語または英熟語を本文から選び出して書き込み，また発音しなさい（動詞は原形を記入しなさい）。

	Japanese	English		Japanese	English
1	痴呆		4	老人性の	
2	痴呆性の		5	脳血管性	
3	症状・病気		6	血管性疾患	

Notes :
cholinesterase inhibitors「コリンエステラーゼ阻害剤」
donepezil hydrochloride「塩酸ドネペジル」，ARICEPT「アリセプト」

Chapter 6 Dementious Disorders: Alzheimer's Disease

	Japanese	English		Japanese	English
7	動脈硬化症		27	常染色体	
8	高血圧症		28	病理学的な	
9	虚血性心疾患		29	収縮	
10	高脂血症		30	老人斑	
11	糖尿病		31	大脳皮質	
12	変性		32	沈着	
13	神経細胞		33	大脳	
14	筋強剛		34	疫学的な	
15	振戦		35	発症	
16	姿勢保持反射障害		36	疫学的	
17	無動		37	遅延させる	
18	寡動		38	被害妄想	
19	自律神経症状		39	幻覚	
20	うつ		40	掛け金を頂る第三者	
21	神経生理的な		41	介護支援者	
22	遺伝的な		42	暴力的な	
23	遺伝子		43	徘徊	
24	認知障害		44	不潔な	
25	見当識障害		45	脆弱な	
26	空間認知機能		46	祖先の	

Unit C Genetic Disorders

2．つぎの各文が本文の内容と一致するものにはT(True), 一致しないものにはF(False)を，文末の（　）に記入しなさい。

（1）Cerebrovascular dementia occurs commonly as one of senile dementious ailment.（　）
（2）Some cases of Parkinson's disease can be heritable.（　）
（3）Medicaments are not available to slow down PD.（　）
（4）Pathological traits of AD are: brain tissue atrophy and appearance of the senile plaque in cerebral cortex.（　）
（5）Risks to have AD can be reduced by daily efforts.（　）

3．つぎの日本語の各文を（　）の中の語を用いて英語の文にしなさい（必要があれば単語を適切な形に変換しなさい）。

（1）本章は，痴呆性障害に関して簡潔に概説し，アルツハイマー症について焦点をおいて記述します。(describe, focus, brief, disorder)

（2）血管性疾患は生活習慣に由来することが頻繁にあります。(vascular, lifestyle, custom, originate)

（3）パーキンソン病は老齢に伴い誰にでも起こり得る可能性があります。(risk, aging, progress)

（4）アルツハイマー病は，徐々に進行し，重篤な状態では自律して摂食，着替えや会話ができなくなり，介護者の支援が必須となる。(gradual, require, independent)

Chapter 6　Dementious Disorders: Alzheimer's Disease　　**67**

（5）痴呆性障害をもつ患者は，病状の進行に伴い，被害妄想や幻覚を引き起こしたり，暴言，暴力，徘徊や不潔な行為などの行動をすることがある。（cause, behavior, filty）

4．つぎの各問いに英語で答えなさい。

（1）How should we care the patients with dementia?

（2）How do we reduce the risk to dementious disorders?

（3）How medicaments help coping with the AD?

（4）What are the general appearance symptoms of PD?

（5）Can we expect the future medical research could alleviate the various aspects of the medication on and cares for dementia?

Chapter 7 Chromosomal Disorders

Chromosomal disorders occur in any higher organisms. Two major categories are polyploidy and anueploidy. Also relatively minor aberrant events are deletion, duplication, inversion, and translocation on the local region of a chromosome.

Small changes could occur at DNA aliments of any organisms during the replication processes by miss-leading the template DNA information of which make genetic information as to be genes, which consequently relate to the hereditary traits. But such a minor error of DNA replication could often be self-repaired by internal mechanisms to keep the hereditary information stable. However, when DNAs are exposed to excess alteration pressure such as chemical mutagens and irradiation, the irreversible change can take place, ending to mutation. These sort of the alternation changes the genetic information consequently gene function which are vital to fundamental physiological reaction(s) of human bodies, ending to illness.

In this chapter, focus is made on the aneuploidy and their association with hereditary ailments which makes dysfunction to the human. The genetic disorders caused at the gene level should be explained more at Chapter 8, including pathogensis-related genes and heritable diseases.

Plants can have a variety of minor to major chromosomal aberrations. Polyploidy is the common occurrence in Plant Kingdom. And it is natural for many species: even the half of the angiosperms, which contain quarter millions of species, can be regarded as polyploidy or

Notes :

dysfunction「不全」, angiosperms「被子植物」

originated from polyploidization. However, there is rare occurrence of polyploidy in mammalians, and it is regarded as unusual except for some extraordinary cases such in rodents.

Aneuploidy is general term in the addition or deletion of an entire chromosome, missing of one chromosome is called monosomy, and an addition of a whole chromosome is designated as trisomy. Those individuals with one missing or additional chromosome are called, monosomics and trisomics, respectively. While it is absolutely rare in mammals, nullisomics is possible in higher plants, which have an absence of a pair of homologous chromosomes, which means an entire chromosome-based genetic information deleted.

Often plants can allow anueploidy conditions and they can survive and produce filial progenies. Even some of unique changes such as trisomics on Datura, rice and wheat, have been employed for genetic study of the gene doses and the role of chromosomes and their association with specific loci at classical plant cytogenetics. However, in the case of mammalians such chromosomal abnormalities could be fatal at gametic or embryonic stages, or cause significant functional disadvantages at and after birth.

Cause of the aneuploidy is mainly attributed to abnormal chromosome separation either at mitosis or meiosis. Nondisjunction is the direct explanation, and it is the failure of the chromosome segregation in the mitosis or meiosis. The nondisjunction happens by chance, but it increases the frequency by interference with microtubule polymerization action at molecular biological studies in many cases. Such events could be natural occurrence by more exposures to chemical

Notes :
rodents「げっ歯類」．filial「後代の」．Datura「チョウセンアサガオ属」
microtubule polymerization「紡錘糸重合」

mutagens, radiation and extraordinary temperatures, and also with malnutrition in case of the meiosis. Meiotic divisions are more vulnerable to the nondisjunction.

Viable monosomy can occur in human, but death reaches in utero on the monosomics in any human autosomes. Turner Syndrome is the result of monosomy on human X chromosome. The probability of the syndrome is one out of 5,000 female births. The disadvantage of the syndrome is that surviving females are, sterile due to rudimentary ovaries and gonadal streak, constriction of aorta, extraordinary short stature, elbow deformity etc.. The intelligence level is about normal, while there may be some cognitive functional pitfalls.

Klinefelter syndrome and Down syndrome are caused by the trisomy. Those occurrences are not so low: one out of one thousand births could be such a possibility.

Klinefelter syndrome is caused by an addition of X chromosomes to male gender with XXY, with testicular insufficiency as general observation. Also variants by tetrasomy (XXXY, XXYY) and pentasomy (XXXXY), are possible on the syndrome. Persons with such extra chromosome(s) are lanky build, sterile, more chance to osteoporosis, and some mentally retardant with slightly feminized physical appearance including breast development. However, males with XYY condition, is fertile.

Down Syndrome is caused by Chromosome 21 trisomy. The abnormalities come different degree of mental retardance and some physical weakness. Males with the syndrome do not reproduce fertile

Notes :
Turner Syndrome「ターナー症候群」
Klinefelter syndrome「クラインフェルター症候群」
Down syndrome「ダウン症候群」, lanky「やせ気味の」

gamete, but female with the ailment could have functional gamete and produce normal and trisomic progeny. Occurrence of Down syndrome is often attributed to the maternal age, and relatively older mothers could have higher risk of having trisomy. Trisomy can occur at the family with no history of such patients, and also some specific case with low chance is associated with hereditary matters with chromosomal translocation. Statistically, it could happen at the frequency of one out of 1,500 births. Unfortunately, many of the individuals with the Down syndrome live only to the average of seventeen years old, and only less than 10 % of the persons could survive beyond age of 40 years.

Aneuploid is often deleterious due to the imbalance in genome, and consequently effects on the function and behavior of the individuals with aneuploidy. But, again, readers should be aware that those such chromosomal disorders can occur to any family, and victims are very vulnerable and need care with consideration.

Exercises

1. つぎの 1 ～ 43 の語に対応する英単語または英熟語を本文から選び出して書き込み，また発音しなさい（動詞は原形を記入しなさい）。

	Japanese	English		Japanese	English
1	染色体		7	重複	
2	3染色体		8	逆位	
3	遺伝的な / 遺伝		9	転座	
4	遺伝的な / 遺伝学		10	異常	
5	異数体 / 異数性		11	倍数性	
6	欠失		12	倍数化	

Unit C　Genetic Disorders

	Japanese	English		Japanese	English
13	1染色体性		29	未発達な卵巣	
14	3染色体性		30	性腺(精巣や卵巣)形成不全	
15	1染色体		31	不妊	
16	零染色体		32	緊縮／くびれ	
17	細胞遺伝学		33	大動脈	
18	致命的な		34	欠陥	
19	配偶子の／配偶子		35	精巣機能不全症	
20	胚の／胚		36	4染色体性	
21	不分離		37	5染色体性	
22	体細胞分裂		38	骨粗鬆症	
23	減数分裂		39	遅延した	
24	化学突然変異源		40	生殖する	
25	栄養不良		41	繁殖力のある	
26	障害		42	不均衡	
27	子宮		43	脆弱な	
28	常染色体				

2．つぎの各文が本文の内容と一致するものにはT(True)，一致しないものにはF(False)を，文末の（　）に記入しなさい。

（1）Chromosomal disorders are not deleterious in human. (　　)

（2）Aneuploidy is the same as polyploidy. (　　)

（3）Deletion, duplication and inversion are minor abnormalities on a chromosome. (　　)

（4）Occurrence of human aneuploidy is less than natural mutation frequency. (　　)

（ 5 ）Both polyploidy and aneuploidy can be seen commonly in higher plants. (   )

3. つぎの日本語の各文を（   ）の中の語を用いて英語の文にしなさい（必要があれば単語を適切な形に変換しなさい）。
（ 1 ）染色体異常は高等生物で一般的にみられる（higher organisms, observe）

（ 2 ）遺伝的な異常については，多様な遺伝的因子が関連しており，染色体異常も主要な範ちゅうに入る。（associate, category, factor）

（ 3 ）植物では，倍数性や異数性は一般的にみられる。倍数体は，被子植物では自然界で一般的にみられる。

（ 4 ）ほ乳類での染色体異常は，一般的には配偶子あるいは胚形成時で致死になる。（fatal, mammalians）

（ 5 ）染色体不分離は，偶然に起こり得る。（by chance, nondisjunction, happen）

Unit C　Genetic Disorders

4．つぎの各問いに英文で答えなさい。

（ 1 ） What would cause higher chances on the chromosomal nondisjunction?

（ 2 ） What is Turner syndrome?

（ 3 ） What is the general observation on the Klinfelter syndorome?

（ 4 ） Which autosome has association with Down syndrome?

（ 5 ） Would the chromosomal disorders occur only in occasion with specific groups of people?

Chapter 8   Hereditary Diseases and Gene Therapy

Hereditary disorders are commonly known. By traditional knowledge, many societies have avoided marriages with families having historical records on certain categories of illness.

Many of hereditary diseases have been studied in the history of medical sciences, especially the human genome research opened very broad opportunities to comprehend the genetics of the human ailments. The cause, mechanisms, occurrence, syndromes and potential prevention have been examined to cope with such categories of illness. For examples, cancers, dementious disorders, immunological dysfunctions, are often associated with genetic disorders.

The cause of the genetic disease could be a minor alteration of a locus by a mutation based on deletion, substitution and/or insertion of nucleic acids or DNA. A typical example is the sickle cell anemia: the result of a failure of hemoglobin molecules leads to dysfunction of the blood cells and anemia. This is controlled by a locus and normal and sickle allele are codominant. Only one nucleic acid changes the function: at normal allele corresponding nucleic acid aliment is CCTGaGGAG but with sickle cell allele, CCTGtGGAG, thus change of A to T makes the genetic cause for the illness. The difference can be detected by the combination of molecular biology approaches: PCR of the locus followed by *Mst*II restriction enzyme digest, which is called CAPS technique. The difference of allele product is only one amino

---

Notes :
PCR: polymerase chain reaction 「試験管内遺伝子増幅」
*Mst*II restriction enzyme 「制限酵素の一種」
CAPS: Clevaged Amplified Polymorphic Site

acid: replacement of glutamic acid to valine makes the sickle cell allele product. The disease is common in African and African Americans, and on the latter case the chance of incidence of the disease is one out of 625 individuals.

Some of chromosome linked genetic disorders are historically well known as text models. Hemophilia, bleeders disease, is incompletion or failing of blood clotting and it is controlled by recessive sex-linked inheritance on X chromosome. Hypophosphatemia is vitamin D resistant rickets as a dominant trait also on X chromosome. Cystic fibrosis occurs with high probability among Caucasians with one person over 2,000 individuals. The disease is associated with recessive allele on Chromosome 7, which shows defective cell membrane proteins, excessive mucus production, digestive and respiratory failure.

Huntington's disease is caused by a dominant allele on chromosome Ⅳ. A quotation is made from Hereditary Foundation on Huntington's disease (http://www.hdfoundation.org/home.php): a fatal, autosomal-dominant neurological illness causing involuntary movements, severe emotional disturbance and cognitive decline. Huntington's disease usually strikes in mid-life, in the thirties or forties, although it can also attack children and the elderly. There is no treatment to halt the inexorable progression, which leads to death after ten to twenty-five years. Because it is an autosomal-dominant disorder, each child of a parent with Huntington's disease has a 50 % risk of inheriting the illness. In the United States, the prevalence of the disease is about 10 cases per 100,000 people — about 30,000 people in all. There are another 150,000 individuals at risk.

Notes :
gutamic acid「グルタミン酸」, valine「バリン」
Huntington's disease「ハンチントン舞踏病」

Chapter 8 Hereditary Diseases and Gene Therapy

Can Hereditary Diseases be Avoided?

In many cases, they are unavoidable unfortunately, but reducing the effects are possible to cope with the hardships caused by the sickness as the occurrence of disease can be predicted from the hereditary background and medical diagnosis. Also prior knowledge and preventive efforts on the expression of sickness reduce risks of disease occurrence, so that caring own life style is also another consideration to be prepared for incidents.

A challenge to change the destiny: Gene therapy is the genetic engineering method to alter the genetic nature by inserting a gene fragment into human genome for changing the function of the target disease-causing gene(s) to reduce or eliminate the disease. Namely, it is a transgenic technology.

Cystic fibrosis can be the example: the gene causing the disease has been studied and isolated, so that with the genomic information and genetic engineering tools, normal gene counterpart could be replaced with the abnormal one to cure the disease in the patients. This is a somatic gene therapy, and in practice for the cystic fibrosis, the wild-type normal gene is introduced into lung cells of a patient. Practically, this is the same as drug administered into the specific affected tissue or organ. However, the genetic cure by the somatic gene therapy results only on the somatic cells of the patient with the therapy, but not to the filial progenies.

Consideration: Ethical considerations should be made on handling the genetic information of individuals as in the last chapter of this book. The information could be used for various social activities such as rating of health insurances, employments and marriages. Prejudice and unfair actions must not be received at any occasion on the hereditary disease possibilities as it

Unit C　Genetic Disorders

could happen to everybody, even sometimes with very high chance such on cystic fibrosis on Caucasians, and also as like other diseases caused by different reasons, patients are very vulnerable and must be cared.

Exercises

1. つぎの 1 〜 37 の語に対応する英単語または英熟語を本文から選び出して書き込み，また発音しなさい（動詞は原形を記入しなさい）。

	Japanese	English		Japanese	English
1	ゲノム		16	対立遺伝子	
2	発生		17	血液凝固	
3	免疫不全		18	血友病	
4	変化/改変		19	出血する	
5	遺伝子座		20	劣性	
6	突然変異		21	低リン血症	
7	欠失		22	優性	
8	置換		23	くる病	
9	挿入/添加		24	嚢胞性線維症	
10	核酸		25	可能性/確立	
11	鎌形赤血球症		26	粘液	
12	ヘモグロビン		27	失敗/衰退	
13	分子		28	致命的な	
14	共優性		29	遺伝子工学	
15	制限酵素		30	遺伝子組換えの	

Chapter 8 Hereditary Diseases and Gene Therapy

	Japanese	English		Japanese	English
31	体細胞の		35	保険	
32	投与する		36	雇用	
33	倫理（学）		37	脆弱な	
34	偏見				

2. つぎの各文が本文の内容と一致するものにはT(True)，一致しないものにはF(False)を，文末の（　）に記入しなさい。

（1）Male bold head is the infectious disease rather than hereditary possibilities. （　）

（2）Sickle cell anemia does not have major damage to daily activities. （　）

（3）All hereditary diseases are associated with sex linked traits. （　）

（4）Cystic fibrosis could occur with a high chance in a specific population such on caucasians. （　）

（5）All genetic diorders cannot be cured. （　）

3. つぎの日本語の各文を（　）の中の語を用いて英語の文にしなさい（必要があれば単語を適切な形に変換しなさい）。

（1）ハンチントン舞踏病は致命的な病である。この病気は，常染色体で優性遺伝を行い神経障害を起こす。奇異な動作，感情の不安定，認知能力の退行などがみられる。(autosomal, cognitive, fatal)

Unit C　Genetic Disorders

（2）血友病は，血液凝固について不完全か凝固しないような状態であり，これはX染色体上の劣性遺伝子によって伴性遺伝する。

（3）遺伝子治療は，標的となる疾病原因の遺伝子の機能を，外部からのヒトゲノムへの遺伝子断片の挿入によって改変し，病害を減退あるいは無効化する遺伝子工学手法である。(gene therapy, insert, reduce, eliminate)

（4）本書最後の章で記述があるように，個人の遺伝情報の取扱いについて，倫理的な配慮を行うべきである。(handle, ethics, describe)

（5）正常と病気に関わる対立遺伝子の違いは，分子生物学的手法を組み合わせることによって検出できる。(detection, molecular biology, abnormal)

4．つぎの各問いに英語で答えなさい。
（1）すべての人はなんらかの遺伝病をもっている可能性を否定できない。

（2）囊胞性線維症，低リン血症による障害や血友病は，すべて遺伝病である。一方，現在医科学によって原因や関連遺伝子の研究が促進され，対処法も多様に解明されてきている。

（3）遺伝病の原因は，核酸つまりDNAの欠失，置換や挿入などの突然変異によって起こる一遺伝子座の微小な変異によることもある。

（4）ハンチントン病は，4番の常染色体に座乗する優性遺伝子に起因する。

（5）個人の遺伝情報は，人間社会で多様な用途で使われる可能性があるが，倫理的な側面は十分に配慮されなければならない。

Unit D　Future in Multidisciplinary Medical Technology

Chapter 9　Cells, Totipotency and Organogenesis

Stem cells are not only units of biological organization, responsible for the development and the regeneration of tissue and organ systems, but also are units in evolution by natural selection. Stem cells are generally defined as clonogenic cells capable of both self-renewal and multilineage differentiation. Two subsets of stem cells are divided: Long-term subset and short-term subset. The long term subset self-renews for the life of the host, while the short-term subset retains self-renewal capability for a defined interval. The short-term subset can differentiate into multipotent progenitors, which have the ability to differentiate into oligolineage progenitors and utilimately give rise to differentiated progeny. Each stage of differentiation involves functionally irreversible maturation steps.

　　Hematopoietic stem cells (HSCs) are probably the best characterized stem cell population. In the mouse, hematopoiesis occurs by 8 days postconception in the yolk sac blood islands, and the yolk sac vasculature connects via the umbilical vein to the fetal liver. Yolk sac HSCs provide local hematopoiesis during development and participate in lifelong hematopoiessis in the bone marrow, presumably by a natu-

Notes :
clonogenic cells「遺伝群細胞」, multipotent progenitors「多型潜在性先駆体」
oligolineage progenitors「多型分化先駆体」
hematopoietic stem cells (HSCs)「造血幹細胞」
hematopoiesis「造血，血液新生」, umbilical vein「臍(さい)静脈」
bone marrow「骨髄」

ral migration of HSCs from one hematopoitic microenvironment to the other. At least two successive mobilizations of HSCs occur — from the embryonic loci to fetal liver, and from fetal liver to spleen and bone marrow. These movements are genetically controlled in part via changes in expression of cell surface adhesion molecules (**Figure 9.1**).

Understanding the biology of HSCs has led to a number of medical advances in cancer therapy, transplantation, and autoimmunity.

Long-term stem cells

Short-term stem cells

Multipotent progenitors

Oligolineage progenitors

Differentiated progency

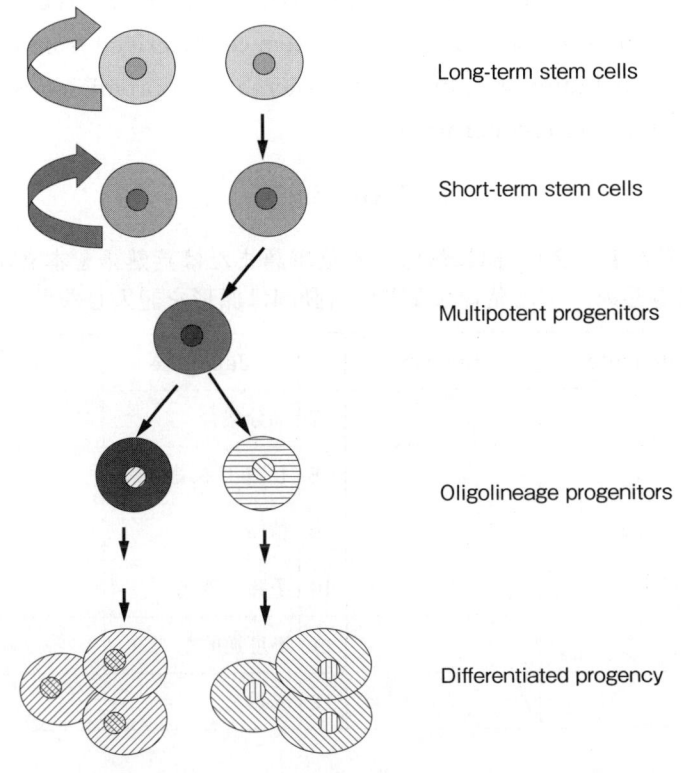

Figure 9.1 Hematopoietic stem cells (HSCs)

Notes :
embryonic loci「胚座」, adhesion molecules「接着分子」

Unit D Future in Multidisciplinary Medical Technology

The regeneration of the haematolymphoid system following an otherwise lethal dose of whole-body irradiation or chemotherapy became the basis for the use of bone marrow transplantation.

Stem cells other than HSCs in mammalian somatic tissue are found capable of generating somatic cell systems such as the central nervous system (CNS) and organ system. Human fetal clonogenic CNS neurosphere-initiating cells have been proved to undergo multi-linage differentiation, which are expected to regenerate regions of the brain with appropriate connections. Stem cells derived from primitive endoderm, including gut, liver and pancreas are promising to the application of organ regeneration.

Exercise

1. つぎの1～29の語に対応する英単語または英熟語を本文から選び出して書き込み，また発音しなさい（動詞は原形を記入しなさい）。

	Japanese	English		Japanese	English
1	再生		7	部分集合	
2	進化（論）		8	もち続ける，維持する	
3	能力がある		9	結局	
4	自己再生		10	子孫，後代	
5	多系		11	不可逆的な	
6	分化		12	成熟	

Notes:

haematolymphoid system 「造血リンパ系」

central nervous system (CNS) 「中枢神経系」

neurosphere-initiating cells 「神経球開始細胞」, endoderm 「内胚葉」

	Japanese	English		Japanese	English
13	特性，特徴		22	移植手術	
14	妊娠後，受胎後		23	自己免疫	
15	卵黄嚢		24	致死（線）量	
16	脈管構造		25	放射線照射	
17	推定されるように		26	化学療法	
18	移動		27	ほ乳類の	
19	微小環境		28	体細胞	
20	継続的な，連続的な		29	最初の，初期の	
21	流通，流動化				

2. つぎの各文が本文の内容と一致するものにはT(True)，一致しないものにはF(False)を，文末の（　）に記入しなさい。

（1）Stem cells is not useful to the regeneration of tissue. (　)

（2）The short term subset of stem cell can retain self-renewal capability for a limited interval. (　)

（3）Hematopoietic stem cells occur in the yolk sac firstly and then move to spleen and bone marrow through liver. (　)

（4）Bone marrow transplantation requires a procedure of lethal dose of whole-body irradiation or chemotherapy. (　)

（5）Hematopoietic stem cells can generate central nervous system. (　)

3. つぎの日本語の各文を（　）の中の語を用いて英語の文にしなさい（必要があれば単語を適切な形に変換しなさい）。

（1）幹細胞は組織や臓器の発生・再生を司る生物的単位だけではなく，自然選択により進化する単位でもある。(development, regeneration, tissue, organ, responsible, evolution）

（2）分化の各時期は機能的に不可逆な成熟ステップに関係する。(differentiation, involve, functionally, maturation, irreversible)

（3）血球幹細胞は幹細胞群の中でいちばん定性されたものであろう。(characterize, population)

（4）血球幹細胞の生物学を理解することは，がん治療，移植と自己免疫のいくつかの医学的な進歩をリードすることになる。(biology, cancer therapy, transplantation, autoimmunity)

（5）血球幹細胞以外のほ乳動物体組織幹細胞は，体のシステムを形成できることがわかった。(mammalian, somatic, generate)

Chapter 9   Cells, Totipotency and Organogenesis

4. つぎの各問いに英語で答えなさい。

(1) Describe the two main properties of stem cells.

(2) How do the stem cells give rise to differentiated progeny?

(3) Where is the first location hematopoiesis occurs in mouse? And how does it connect to liver ?

(4) What is the factor that may control the movement of HSC from embryonic to fetal liver?

(5) What kinds of cells are candidates for the application of organ regeneration?

Chapter 10 Xeno-Transplanting and Substitutive Artificial Parts

Organ transplantation was one of the first methods to restore from and function in modern medicine. In 1955, Murray performed the first successful organ transplant (kidney), and in the early 1960's, he performed the first allogeneic kidney transplantation from a genetically dissimilar donor into an unrelated recipient. As one of the first procedures to overcome the immunologic barrier, this revolutionary procedure marked the modern era in which transplantation could be used as means of therapy for diseased and injured organs.

However, despite the advances in transplantation over the past 50 years, a severe shortage of donor organs limits the availability of this treatment. This has spawned the search for alternative therapies, such as therapeutic cloning and tissue engineering (**Figure 10.1**).

Therapeutic cloning is used to generate early stage embryos that are explanted in culture to produce embryonic stem cell lines whose genetic material is identical to that of its source. These autologous stem cells have the potential to become almost any type of cell in the adult body, and thus would be useful in tissue and organ replacement application. However, banned in most countries for human applications, embryonic stem cells are not adopted clinically.

Most current strategies for tissue/organ replacement is tissue engineering. The strategies generally fall into two categories: acellular matrices and matrices with cells. Acellular tissue matrices are usually prepared by removing cellular components from tissues via mechanical and chemical manipulation to produce collagen-rich matrices.

Note :

organ transplantation「臓器移植」

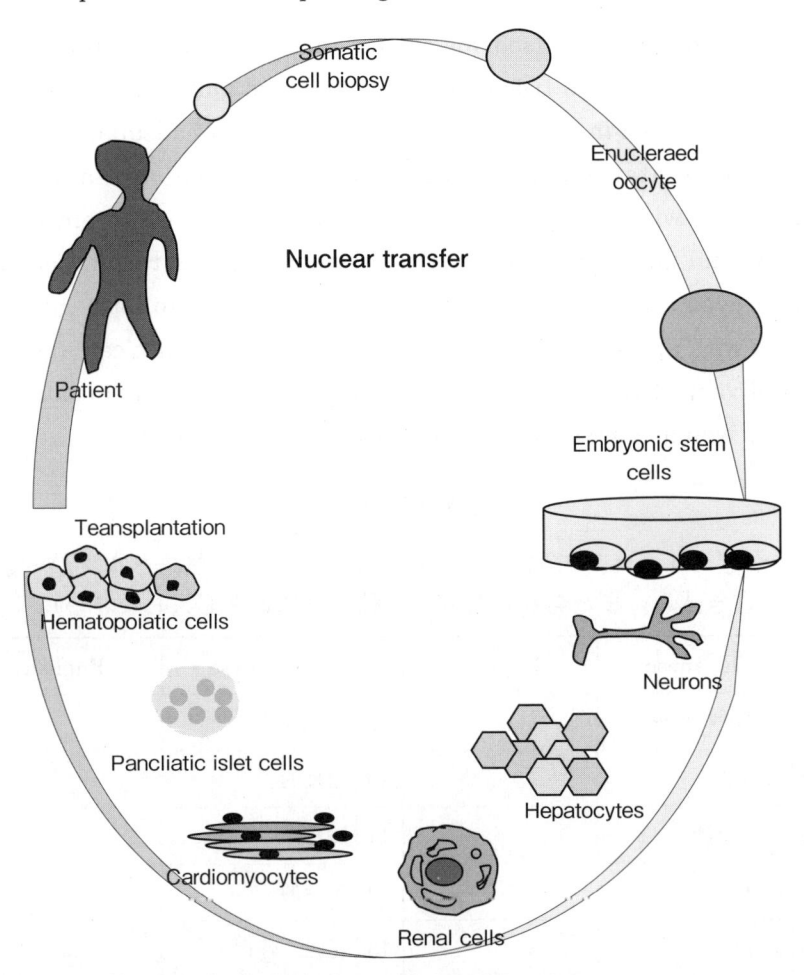

Chapter 10 Xeno-Transplanting and Substitutive Artificial Parts   89

Figure 10.1 Tissue engineering

These matrices tend to slowly degrade on implantation and are generally replaced by the extracelluar matrix (ECM) proteins that are selected by the growing cells.

Note :
extracelluar matrix (ECM)「細胞間質（matrix）の複数形」

90　Unit D　Future in Multidisciplinary Medical Technology

When cells are used for tissue engineering, a small piece of donor tissue or cloned tissue is dissociated into individual cells which are then cultured *in vitro* for sufficient expansion of adequate number. For transplantation, the expand cells are seeded onto a scaffold synthesized with the appropriate biomaterials which can replicate the biologic and mechanical function of native ECM. As a result, biomaterials proved a three-dimensional space for the cells to form into new tissues with appropriate structure and function, and also can allow for the delivery of cells and bioactive factors such as cell adhesion peptides as well as growth factors to desired sites in the body.

Exercise

1．つぎの1～47の語に対応する英単語または英熟語を本文から選び出して書き込み，また発音しなさい（動詞は原形を記入しなさい）。

	Japanese	English		Japanese	English
1	元に戻す，回復する		9	克服する	
2	実行する		10	免疫的	
3	移植組織		11	障害	
4	同種		12	革命的	
5	遺伝学的に		13	紀元，時代	
6	異なる		14	治療	
7	関係ない		15	負傷した	
8	臓器移植者		16	不足	

Notes：
scaffold「足場」，three-dimensional space「立体」
cell adhesion peptides「接着性ペプチド」，growth factors「成長因子」

Chapter 10　Xeno-Transplanting and Substitutive Artificial Parts

	Japanese	English		Japanese	English
17	使用できること		33	操作	
18	処置・療法		34	膠原の豊富な	
19	引き起こす，原因を作る		35	退化させる	
20	代わりの		36	細胞外基質	
21	胚		37	内部に生長する	
22	外植される		38	分離する	
23	幹細胞		39	培養された	
24	同様の		40	培養発展	
25	交換		41	十分な	
26	禁止する		42	播種された	
27	臨床的に		43	合成する	
28	方法，方策		44	複製する	
29	無細胞の		45	生体適応素材	
30	細胞の		46	引き渡し	
31	構成要素		47	生物活性	
32	機械的な				

2．つぎの各文が本文の内容と一致するものには T(True)，一致しないものには F(False) を，文末の（　）に記入しなさい。

（1）The first successful organ transplant is liver.（　）

（2）Immunologic barrier does not exist in allogeneic kidney transplantation.（　）

（3）The use of embryonic stem cells for tissue and organ replace-

ment are banned in a few countries. (　　)
(4) Tissue engineering strategy requires matrices and cells. (　　)
(5) A synthesized scaffold can replicate native ECM when cells are seeded thereon. (　　)

3．つぎの日本語の各文を（　　）の中の語を用いて英語の文にしなさい（必要があれば単語を適切な形に変換しなさい）。
(1) 臓器移植は現代医学による健康回復と臓器を機能化する最初の方法の一つである。(organ, transplantation, restore, function, modern, medicine)

(2) 医療クローニングは，初期胚を生成するために使う。この初期胚を培養組織に移植して胚幹細胞株を樹立するわけである。(therapeutic cloning, embryos, stem cell line, explant, early stage, tissue culture)

(3) 自家幹細胞は成体のほとんどすべての細胞になる可能性をもつ。(autologous, potential, adult body)

(4) 組織・臓器の代替法において最新の方法は組織工学である。(replacement, current, strategy, tissue engineering)

Chapter 10 Xeno-Transplanting and Substitutive Artificial Parts

（５）小さなドナーの組織あるいはクローンした組織から個別細胞を分離してから，生体外で培養し十分の量になるまで増幅する。(donor tissue, cloned tissue, dissociate, individual, in vitro, expansion)

4．つぎの各問いに英語で答えなさい。
（１）What is allogenieic organ transplantation ?

（２）Why cannot the transplantation become a satisfactory treatment?

（３）What are the therapies developed to replace organ transplantation?

（４）How are acellular tissue matrices prepared?

（５）What is the procedure of tissue engineering for transplantation?

Chapter 11 Nano-Medical Technology and Master-Mind Physicians' Skills

Nanotechnology involves the precise manipulation and control of atoms and molecules to create novel materials with properties controlled at the nanoscale, billionths of a meter. Broadly, two production approaches exist; the bottom-up and the top-down.

The bottom-up approach involves physically manipulating small numbers of individual atoms or more complex molecules into structures typically using minute probes. It is possible to push atoms into a desired location using atomically fine force microscope tips, intricately carve material using beams of electrons or heavy metal ions. At present this technology is limited to low-volume, high-performance hipe manufacture. The top-down approach involves controlling physical processes, for example, the conditions under which materials are grown, to coerce atoms and molecules to move themselves as a unit to a desired location or structure. Both approaches can work within both biological and nonbiological systems, bridging important divides between the biological and nonbiological worlds.

A broad range of world-class capabilities have been built covering areas as diverse as nanotubes and composites, superconductors, organic and carbon nanostructures, nanophotonics, nanofabrication in silicon, and organic materials; this extends also to various aspects of health care, especially the low-cost diagnostics and novel drug deliv-

Notes:
atomically fine force microscope tips「原子間力顕微鏡チップ」
beams of electrons「電子ビーム」, high-performance「高性能の」
a broad range of「多様な」, nanophotonics「ナノスケールの光子学」
nanofabrication「ナノスケールで組み立てる」

ery systems. Some of the deliverables in the general area of nanomedicine are: real-space images of biomolecules, label-free rapid protein and DNA diagnostics, individually tailed drugs and selective delivery systems, tracers for food, pharmaceutical, and petrochemical industries, biocompatible scaffolds for tissue engineering, and mobile network-based health care (**Figure 11.1**).

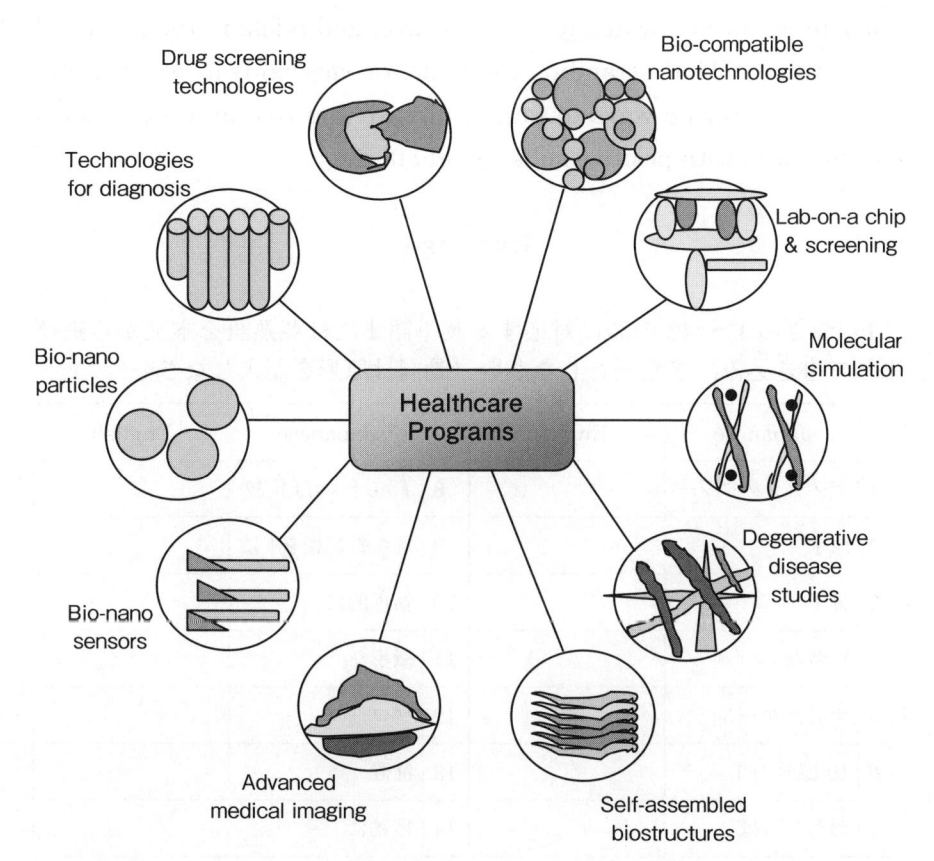

Figure 11.1　The London Center for Nanotechnology has a wide range of bio-nanotechnology and health care research programs.

Notes:
drug delivery systems 「薬物分配システム」, tailed drugs 「作り合わせの薬」

Unit D Future in Multidisciplinary Medical Technology

The cause of therapy for many diseases lies in a greater understanding of the structure and function of proteins. Nanotechnology brings a powerful toolkit to medicine, allowing us to understand the processes driving protein formation and operation. Diseases such as Alzheimer's and Parkinson's disease have been linked to misfolded proteins. Screening chips and atomic force microscopy can be used to grasp proteins, and watch proteins unravel and refold in their natural environments. Understanding fundamental mechanisms of such processes may provide ways to inhibit disease and free up thousands of hospital beds with positive subsequent effects.

Exercise

1. つぎの1～43の語に対応する英単語または英熟語を本文から選び出して書き込み，また発音しなさい（動詞は原形を記入しなさい）。

	Japanese	English		Japanese	English
1	ナノテクノロジー		8	下から上への, 上昇型の	
2	原子		9	逆さまに, 頭を下に	
3	分子		10	物理的に	
4	斬新な		11	微小な	
5	ナノスケール		12	プローブ	
6	10億分の1		13	位置	
7	おおざっぱに		14	複雑に	

Notes：
Alzheimer's disease「アルツハイマー病」
Parkinson's disease「パーキンソン病」
screening chips「スクリーニングチップ」

Chapter 11 Nano-Medical Technology and Master-Mind Physicians' Skills

	Japanese	English		Japanese	English
15	切り分ける		30	標識なし	
16	重金属		31	診断学	
17	注射針		32	追跡子	
18	強制する		33	製薬の	
19	乗り越える		34	石油化学製品	
20	能力，可能性		35	生物学的適合性の	
21	多種多様の		36	工具一式	
22	ナノチューブ		37	折り畳み間違い	
23	超伝導体		38	つかむ，握る	
24	有機の		39	解く	
25	炭素		40	折り畳んだ状態に戻す	
26	シリコン		41	基本の	
27	有機物質		42	抑制する	
28	提出物		43	空ける	
29	真空間の				

2．つぎの各文が本文の内容と一致するものにはT(True)，一致しないものにはF(False)を，文末の（　）に記入しなさい。

（1）The approach using minute process to manipulate small numbers of atoms or complex molecules into structure is called bottom-up approach. （　）

（2）The top-down approach is a process which can control materials growing or can move materials to a desired location. （　）

（3）At present, nanotechnology mainly covers diverse areas of superconductors and carbon nanostructure. （　）
（4）Nanomedicine is not a novel area extended in nanotechnology. （　）
（5）Alzheimer's and Parkinson's diseases are caused by protein misfolding. （　）
（6）Nanotechnology can be used to inhibit disease. （　）

3．つぎの日本語の各文を（　）の中の語を用いて英語の文にしなさい（必要があれば単語を適切な形に変換しなさい）。
（1）原子間微細力顕微鏡のチップを用い，原子を所定の場所に押し付けることは可能である。(atom, desire, location, atomically fine force microscope)

（2）今日，新しいナノテクノロジーは生物的世界と非生物的世界を結びつけた。(nanotechnology, bridge, nonbiological)

（3）超伝導や炭素のナノ構造分野などの技術はすでに確立された。(cover, superconductors, carbon nanostructure)

（4）ナノテクノロジーは医療分野，特に低価格の診断と新たな創薬システムにまでに展開した。(extend, aspect, health care, diagnostics, drug delivery system)

（5）病気原因の探索は，蛋白質の構造と機能をさらに理解することに依存する。(cause, disease, understanding, function, protein)

4．つぎの各問いに英語で答えなさい。
（1）What is nanotechnology?

（2）What is the difference between bottom-up and top-down approach of nanotechnology?

（3）What is the aspect to which nanotechnology extends?

（4）Exemplify the deliverables in the area of nanomedicine.

（5）How can nanotechnology help the therapy of Alzheimer's disease?

Chapter 12 Machine-Aided System

Robot heroes and heroines in science fiction movies and cartoons like Star Wars in US and Astro Boy in Japan have attracted us so much which, as a result, has motivated many robotic researchers. These robots, unlike special purpose machines, are able to communicate with us and perform a variety of complex tasks in the real world. However, such kind of robot does not exit in real world.

Recently, cognitive developmental robotics (CDR) has been started, which aims to understand the cognitive developmental processes that an intelligent robot would require and how to realize them in a physical entity. The key aspect of CDR is its design principle. Existing approaches often explicitly implement a control structure in the robot's 'brain' that was derived from a designer's understanding of the robot's physics, while the CDR structure reflects the robot's own process of understanding through interactions with the environment (**Figure 12.1**).

Cognition and development have been the key issues for human intelligence, and recent progress in these disciplines promoted a new area called developmental cognitive neuroscience (DCN), which emerged at the interface between two of the most fundamental questions that challenge mankind. The first one concerns the relation between the mind and the body, and especially between the physical substance of the brain and the mental processes it supports (cognitive neuroscience). The second concerns the origin of the organized biologi-

---

Notes :
cognitive developmental robotics (CDR)「認知性発達ロボット」
developmental cognitive neuroscience (DCN)「発育認知神経科学」

Chapter 12 Machine-Aided System

Environmental digesting issues
Reward function
Fearing schedule
Learning from easy mission
Gradual increase in complexity
Teaching

Embedded structure
Reinforcement learning
Neural oscillator
Recurrent NN
State vector estimation
Imitation

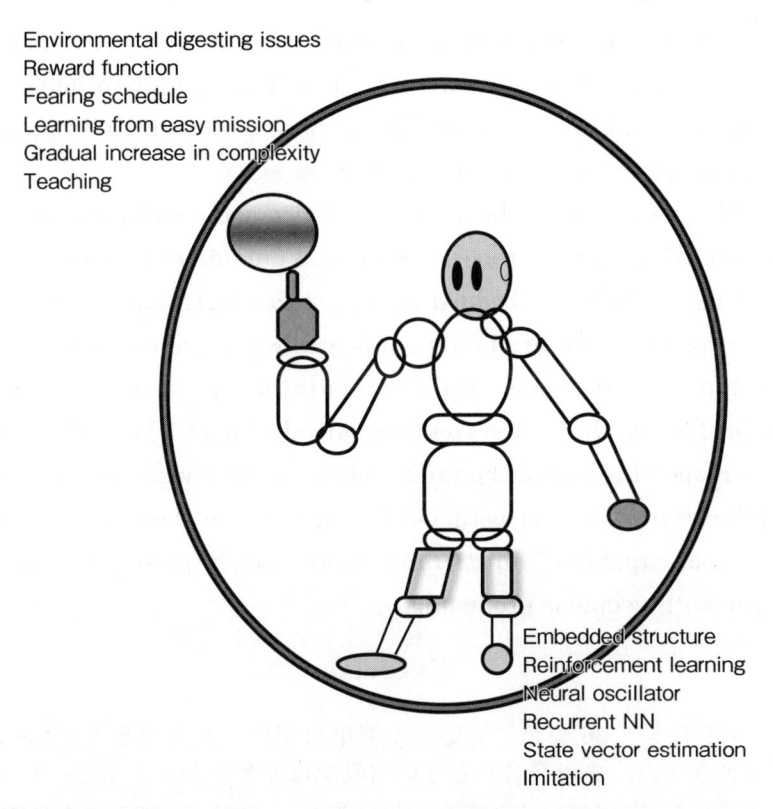

Figure 12.1 Interaction between embedded and environment (modified from Robotics and Autonomous Systems 37, pp.185 ~ 193 (2001))

cal structure such as the highly complex structure of the adult human brain (development).

The difference between CDR and DCN is that CDR is a synthetic or constructive approach with the potential to test its model by implementing them in humanoid robots. The cycle of fault diagnosis and reimplementation may iterate many times in order to refine the mod-

---

Note :

humanoid robots「人型ロボット」

el. This process of refinement is expected to result in a useful model of human interaction. A new way of understanding human beings will develop that differs significantly from the ways in which humans are understood in the natural and social sciences.

The design principle of CDR is that a self-developing structure is embedded inside the robot's brain, and outside environment is set up so that the robot embedded structure can learn and develop from the environment and gradually adapt itself to more complex tasks in more dynamic situations. Environmental design issues include all kinds of factors that come from outside the robot. How other active agents respond is key to the multi-agent learning whether they be cooperative, competitive or both. On the basis of the above design principle, a robot capable of functioning in our society by developing relationship with people is promising.

Exercise

1. つぎの 1 ～ 26 の語に対応する英単語または英熟語を本文から選び出して書き込み，また発音しなさい（動詞は原形を記入しなさい）。

	Japanese	English		Japanese	English
1	英雄的女性		9	相互作用	
2	動機付けられた		10	認知（力）	
3	伝達する		11	中間面	
4	有形の		12	基本の	
5	実体		13	人類	
6	明白に, 明示的に		14	合成の, 総合的な	
7	施行する, 導入する		15	発展的な	
8	物理学, 物理的課程		16	可能な, 可能性のある	

	Japanese	English		Japanese	English
17	分析，判断		22	埋める，組み込む	
18	実行，履行		23	動力学	
19	繰り返す		24	協同の	
20	精製，精錬		25	競争の	
21	意味深く，はっきりと		26	将来有望な	

2．つぎの各文が本文の内容と一致するものにはT(True)，一致しないものにはF(False)を，文末の（　）に記入しなさい。

（1）Traditional robot can communicate with human being. (　)

（2）An intelligent robot does not necessarily need cognitive developmental process to communicate with environment. (　)

（3）Developmental cognitive neuroscience is developed via the disciplines of cognition and development process for robot. (　)

（4）The relation between the mind and the body is related to cognitive neuroscience. (　)

（5）The design principle of CDR is a self-developing structure embedded outside of robot's brain to learn and develop from environment. (　)

3．つぎの日本語の各文を（　）の中の語を用いて英語の文にしなさい（必要があれば単語を適切な形に変換しなさい）。

（1）スターウォーズのような科学フィクション映画と漫画の中のロボット英雄は，現実の世界にはいない。(robot, fiction movie, cartoon, real world)

Unit D　Future in Multidisciplinary Medical Technology

（2）特殊用途機械と違って，映画のロボットは私達と交流できる。(unlike, special purpose, communicate)

（3）最近の進歩で新しい分野の発展性感知脳科学が促進された。(recent, progress, cognitive neuroscience)

（4）モデルを改良するために，間違った診断と再実行のサイクルが何回も繰り返される。(cycle, fault diagnosis, reimplementation, iterate, refine)

（5）この改良プロセスを経て，人間とインタラクションできるようなモデルを作り出せることが期待される。(refinement, result in, usual model, human interaction)

4．つぎの各問いに英語で答えなさい。
（1）Why was cognitive developmental robotics (CDR) started ?

(2) What's the difference of the design principles between existing robot structure and CDR structure?

(3) What is DCN?

(4) What is the design principle of CDR?

(5) What will the intelligent robot learn from the other active agents ?

Chapter 13 Eyes for Blinds: Sensoring Systems

So far, even the most advanced of the experimental devices has provided blind people with only the crudest of black-and-white images, inadequate for navigating unfamiliar surroundings. Most of the artificial eyes currently under development would benefit just the minority of blind people who suffer from diseases such as retinitis pigmentosa (RP) and macular degeneration that degrade retinal cells but leave some of the retina intact. Much farther out are brain-implanted artificial-vision systems that can help people who have lost their eyes in accidents; none of today's devices will work for people who were born blind and whose visual system as a whole remains underdeveloped (**Figure 13.1**).

　　Nevertheless, a combination of improved surgical techniques, miniaturization of electronics, advances in electrode design, and knowledge about how to safely encapsulate electronics in the body are inching the dream of artificial vision closer to reality.

　　Researchers have investigated the use of electricity to stimulate vision for nearly half a century. In the 1960's, a physiologist implanted 80 electrodes on the surface of a blind person's visual cortex, a region at the back of the brain. Wireless stimulation of the electrodes made the patient see spots of light known as phosphenes. This is the first stop for visual signals coming from the eye.

　　By the 1980's, a crop of ophthalmologists began considering a narrower and seemingly easier-to-solve problem: making prostheses

Notes :
retinitis pigmentosa (RP)「網膜色素変性（症）」
retinal cells「網膜細胞」

Chapter 13　Eyes for Blinds: Sensoring Systems

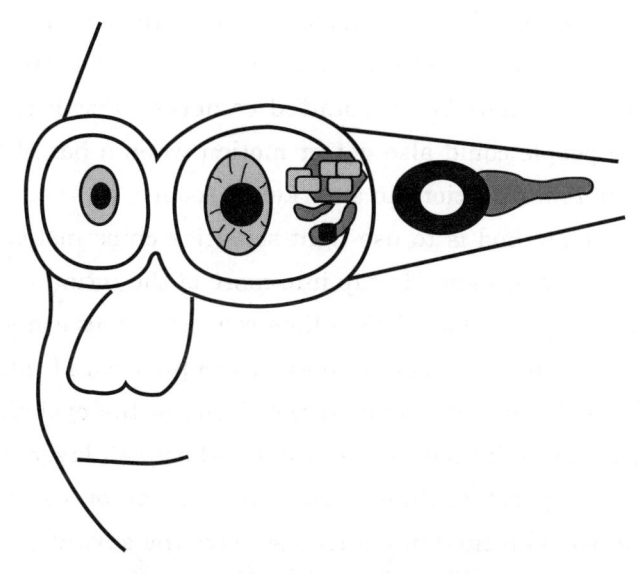

Figure 13.1　A vision for the blind

for the eye. They suggested that degrade photoreceptor cells called rods and cones, still leave large portions of the retina intact even after a patient has become totally blind. The way to stimulate the remaining functional cells was proved feasible in the mid-1990s.

　A device consisting of a tiny video camera perched on the bridge of a pair of glasses, a belt-worn video processing unit, and an electronic box, was developed recently. The electronic box issued to implanted behind the patient's ear that has wires running to a grid of 16 electrodes affixed to the output layer of the retina. The video processor wirelessly transmits a simplified picture of what the camera images to the box, and then the retinal implant stimulates cells in a pattern roughly reflecting that information.

Notes :
　photoreceptor cells「光受容細胞，視細胞」, rods and cones「椎桿体」

After some training with the device, all of the patients could distinguish between the light patterns given off by a plate, cup, and spoon by moving their head-mounted cameras to scan the objects. Some of the people could also detect motion when a bar of light was moved in different directions in a darkened room.

Another method is to use light-sensitive chips instead of camera. The chips are designed to tap into more of the retina's image processing. In the retina, about 125 million rods and cones connect to just 1.2 million optic nerve fibers, a 100-to-1 compression of information. Placing electrodes directly against the lining of the eyeball, enables the electrodes to excite the retina's intermediate cell layers and allow those layers to perform their normal processing of visual signals. These so-called subretinal implants also have the advantage of stimulating the retina in its natural topography. Theoretically, it is provoking more natural perceptions.

Exercise

1. つぎの 1 ~ 38 の語に対応する英単語または英熟語を本文から選び出して書き込み，また発音しなさい（動詞は原形を記入しなさい）。

	Japanese	English		Japanese	English
1	進歩した，新型の		8	少数	
2	実験的な		9	退化させる	
3	器具		10	移植する	
4	品物が良くない		11	自己	
5	不十分な		12	結合	
6	操縦する，誘導する		13	外科手術の	
7	人造の		14	小型化	

Chapter 13 Eyes for Blinds: Sensoring Systems

	Japanese	English		Japanese	English
15	電子工学		27	位置する	
16	電極		28	ベルト付き	
17	カプセルに包む		29	格子	
18	少しずつ動く		30	添付する	
19	生理学者		31	伝送する	
20	皮質		32	識別する	
21	眼内閃光		33	視覚の	
22	眼科医		34	圧縮	
23	外観上		35	中間型	
24	人工器官		36	刺激する	
25	網膜		37	形態（学）	
26	実現可能な		38	理論上	

2. つぎの各文が本文の内容と一致するものにはT(True)，一致しないものにはF(False)を，文末の（　）に記入しなさい。

(1) New visual devices can work for people who were born blind so far. (　)

(2) A combination of surgical and electronic techniques improves artificial vision closer to reality. (　)

(3) Degrade photo receptor cells leave no portions of the retina intact when a patient has become totally blind. (　)

(4) New visual devices is a glasses on which tiny video camera perched. (　)

(5) Light sensitive chips cannot replace video camera because chips cannot tap into more of the retina's image processing. (　)

3. つぎの日本語の各文を（　　）の中の語を用いて英語の文にしなさい（必要があれば単語を適切な形に変換しなさい）。

（1）現在の装置のどちらも生まれつきの盲目者に使えるわけではない。（device, born blind）

（2）研究者達は，半世紀に近いあいだ電気を用いて視覚を刺激することを研究してきた。（researcher, investigate, electricity, stimulate, vision）

（3）電極の無線刺激によって患者は phosphense という光のスポットを見ることができる。（wireless, patient, spot of light, phosphenes）

（4）1990年代半ば，残った機能性細胞を刺激する方法は実行可能であることが証明された。（stimulate, remaining, functional, feasible）

（5）暗室で一束の光を異なる方向に異動させると，何人かの人たちがその動きを見ることができる。（detect, motion, bar, direction, darkened room）

4. つぎの各問いに英語で答えなさい。

(1) To whom do the existing artificial eyes benefit?

(2) What is the limitation of the existing artificial eyes?

(3) What kind of techniques are introduced to the artificial eyes so that the dream of artificial vision closer to reality?

(4) Why did the ophthalmologiests think it is possible to visualize the total blind eyes?

(5) How does the tiny video camera perched on the bridge of glasses work on visualization for the blind people?

Unit E Preventive Medicine and Social Consideration

Chapter 14 Obesity and Exercise

Obesity is now common within the world's population and the prevalence is continually rising. It is beginning to replace malnutrition and infectious diseases as the most significant contributor to ill health. Obesity should no longer be regarded simply as a cosmetic problem affecting certain individuals, but an epidemic that threatens global wellbeing. "Obesity is associated with an increased prevalence of socioeconomic hardship due to a higher rate of disability, early retirement, and widespread discrimination." It was stated by the American Association of Clinical Endocrinologists (AACE) in 1988.

14.1 The Definition of Obesity

The current measurement of obesity is defined by a body-mass index (BMI), weight divide by square of the height kg/m^2. The America Institute for Cancer Research (AICR) considered the classification overweight and obesity as **Table14.1**. Morbid obesity (over 40 kg/m^2), also referred to as clinically severe obesity or extreme obesity, is a chronic disease that afflicts approximately 9 million adult Americans. Central obesity ("apple-shaped" or "abdominal obesity") is when the main deposits of body fat are localized around the abdomen and the upper body. Another diagnose to measurement of obesity is waist-hip ration, when this exceeds 1.0 in men and 0.9 in women. Abdominal obesity is associated most frequently with metabolic syndrome.

Notes:
body-mass index (BMI)「体格指数,肥満度指数」, morbid obesity「病的肥満」

Table 14.1 The America Institute for Cancer Research considered the classification overweight and obesity

BMI*	WHO classification
<18.5	underweight
18.5 – 24.9	health and normal
25.0 – 29.9	overweight
30.0 – 39.9	obesity or obese
>40.0	morbid obesity

*BMI is the weight in kilograms divided by the square of the height in metres.

14.2　Obesity and Disease

In particular, obesity is associated with several medical conditions including: the development of type 2 diabetes mellitus (adult-onset type), insulin resistance, coronary heart disease (CHD) and stroke, high blood pressure (hypertension), an increased incidence of certain forms of cancer (colorectal, renal, breast, esophageal, gastric cardia, and endometrial), gallbladder disease, gallstones, gout, osteoarthritis, and impaired respiratory systems such as respiratory complications (obstructive sleep apnoea). Other afflictions obese individuals are prone to include infertility, birth defects, carpal tunnel syndrome, and

Notes :
adult-onset type「成人発症型」, insulin resistance「インスリン抵抗性」
coronary heart disease (CHD)「冠状動脈性心臓病」, osteoarthritis「変形性関節症」
respiratory complications「呼吸器の鬱血」
obstructive sleep apnoea「閉塞性換気障害，睡眠無呼吸」, infertility「不妊症」
carpal tunnel syndrome「手根管症候群」

liver disease. Also, life-insurance data and epidemiological studies confirm that increasing degrees of overweight and obesity are important predictors of decreased life expectancy.

14.3 Factors to Effect Obesity

Obesity is not a single disorder but a heterogeneous group of conditions with multiple causes. The global epidemic of obesity results from a combination of genetic susceptibility, increased availability of high-energy foods and decreased requirement for physical activity in modern society. Although genetic differences are of undoubted importance, the marked rise in the prevalence of obesity is best explained by behavioral and environmental changes that have resulted from technological advances (**Figure 14.1**).

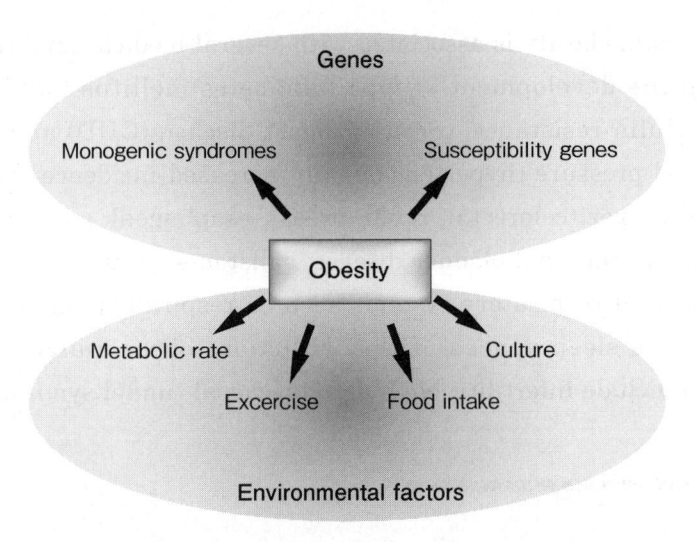

Figure 14.1 Factors influencing the development of obesity (Nature, vol. 404: pp.635-643)

Note:
life expectancy「平均寿命」

Psychological factors also influence eating habits. Eating disorder can lead to obesity, especially binge eating disorder (BED). Many people eat in response to negative emotions such as boredom, sadness, or anger. It is suggested that overweight and obese people are compulsive eaters, anxious, depressed, under stress, or trying to compensate for deficiencies in their lives. Obesity with the most sever binge eating problems are also likely to have symptoms of depression and low self-esteem.

14.4　Treatment of Obesity: Limited Diet and Exercise

The mainstay of treatment for obesity is an energy- limited diet and increased exercise (physical activity). Dietary therapy involves instruction on how to adjust a diet to reduce the number of calories eaten. Reducing calories moderately is essential to achieve a slow but steady weight loss, which is also important for maintenance of weight loss. Strategies of dietary therapy include teaching about calorie content of different foods, food composition (fats, carbohydrates, and proteins), reading nutrition labels, types of foods to buy, and how to prepare foods. The evidence suggests that numerous dietary changes contribute to the reduction in chronic disease risk, including elimination of refined carbohydrates and fatty foods, such as fast food and sugar-containing beverages, and substitution with a diet based largely on whole foods high in fiber and nutrient density.

When the health problems related to overweight and obesity are considered, the decrease in physical activity is also an important factor. People with overweight and obesity have alterations in skeletal

Notes：
binge eating disorder (BED)「過食症」，compulsive eater「過食症の人」
low self-esteem「自尊心の低さ」，mainstay of treatment「治療の柱」
skeletal muscle「骨格筋」

muscle structure and function compared to those who are normal weight that could also contribute to variability in the exercise response. These alterations include a lower percentage of type I and higher percentage of type II muscle fibers, impaired muscle oxidative capacity, a diminished ability to alter fuel utilization between carbohydrate and lipid under conditions of metabolic demand, and increased intramuscular lipid accumulation. In addition, excess adipose tissue releases a variety of neurohormones and cytokines that blunt insulin-stimulated glucose uptake by the muscle. This adiposity-associated structural and metabolic skeletal muscle alterations have been postulated to contribute to the impaired exercise capacity that is sometimes reported in people with overweight and obesity.

Exercise helps people reduce weight, maintain weight, and can help fight obesity. Studies indicated the short-term relative and allometric muscle strength response to resistance training may be attenuated among adults who are overweight and obese. People who are overweight and obese experience numerous health benefits from exercise training programs even in the absence of significant amounts of weight loss. The benefits of exercise in improvement of cardiopulmonary physical fitness and the prevention and treatment of type 2 diabetes mellitus have also been recognized. Type 2 diabetic patients have normal exercise-induced glucose uptake in skeletal muscle. Skeletal muscle is responsible for a major portion of uptake glucose in the postprandial state, mediated by an increase in circulating levels of insulin. The insulin pathway was necessary for glucose uptake in to skeletal muscle. It has become an evident that an alternative pathway exists in which muscle contraction (exercise) is able to stimulate

Notes :
muscle fibers「筋繊維」, cytokines「サイトカイン」

glucose uptake and can thereby bypass muscle insulin resistance. The findings reinforce that the position effect of exercise on insulin sensitivity and for the prevention and treatment of diabetes.

If you are obese, your exercise program should be based on low-intensity aerobic activity where the duration is progressively increased. Duration and frequency are more important than intensity. As long as the increase in energy expenditure is sufficient, low-intensity endurance exercise is likely to generate beneficial metabolic effects that would be essentially similar to those produce by high-intensity exercise. In addition to aerobic activity, you should engage in a weight or resistance training routine. It not only strengths the muscles and bones, but also raises metabolism by increasing the muscle-to-fat ration. As a result, you will burn more calories at rest. Also, your exercise program should include stretching exercises for enhanced flexibility and mobility. Studies suggest that people who have trained for a long time develop more efficient mechanism for burning fat and able to stay leaner.

Exercise improves psychological well-being and replaces sedentary habits that usually lead to snaking. Exercise may even act as a mild appetite suppressant. People who exercise are more apt to stay on a diet plan. Regular exercise (combined with proper nutrition) can conquer the battle against obesity as well as safeguard against the health risks associated with obesity. In fact, research has shown that regular exercise is the common denominator for formerly obese individuals who have kept the weight off for a long period of time. Therefore, please remember to keep regular exercise and do not give up easily.

Notes :
sedentary habits 「座りぐせ」, appetite suppressant 「食欲抑制剤」

Exercises

1. つぎの 1～59 の語に対応する英単語または英熟語を本文から選び出して書き込み，また発音しなさい（動詞は原形を記入しなさい）。

	Japanese	English		Japanese	English
1	肥満症		19	脳梗塞	
2	流行，罹患率		20	高血圧症	
3	栄養不足		21	結腸直腸の	
4	感染症		22	腎臓部の	
5	広範囲に及ぶ		23	食道の	
6	差別		24	胃の噴門	
7	慢性病		25	子宮内膜	
8	伝染病		26	胆嚢	
9	社会経済の		27	胆石	
10	苦境		28	痛風	
11	悩ます		29	～の傾向がある	
12	だいたい		30	疫学的な	
13	腹部の		31	異成分からなる	
14	堆積させる		32	消費	
15	腹部		33	心理的な	
16	胴囲と臀囲の比		34	倦怠，退屈	
17	内臓脂肪症候群		35	補償する	
18	糖尿病		36	欠乏，不足	

Chapter 14　Obesity and Exercise

	Japanese	English		Japanese	English
37	指示		49	心肺の	
38	微細な		50	食後の	
39	置換		51	循環する	
40	変化性，可変性		52	無視する	
41	筋肉内の		53	有酸素活動	
42	蓄積		54	柔軟性	
43	脂肪組織		55	動きやすさ	
44	神経ホルモン		56	〜の傾向がある	
45	鈍くなる		57	克服する	
46	脂肪過多症		58	共通の特徴	
47	前提とする，要求する		59	三日坊主	
48	相対成長の				

2. つぎの各文が本文の内容と一致するものにはT(True)，一致しないものにはF(False)を，文末の（　）に記入しなさい。

（1）Obesity or gaining weight is not only physical but also psychological problems.（　）

（2）Body-mass index (BMI) is the only one measurement to diagnose obesity.（　）

（3）Abdominal obesity is associated most frequently with metabolic syndrome.（　）

（4）Gene susceptibility is an important factor for obesity so this is useless to exercise and limited diet for weight loss.（　）

（5）People with overweight and obesity have alterations in skeletal muscle structure and function compared to those who are normal weight.（　）

3. つぎの日本語の各文を（　）の中の語を用いて英語の文にしなさい（必要があれば単語を適切な形に変換しなさい）。

（1）肥満によって悪い影響を受ける人にとっては，単なる美容の問題として扱うべきではない。肥満は世界中の人々の健康を損うことにつながる。(no longer be regarded…., but)

（2）人は，退屈，悲しみ，怒りといった否定的な感情を紛らすために食べることがある。(in response to)

（3）多くの種類の食物を替えて食べることで慢性疾患になるリスクを減らすことができる。(contribute to, reduction in)

（4）身体のエネルギー消費の増加が十分なとき，短時間の軽い運動で十分な代謝が得られやすい。(as long as, be likely to)

（5）運動する人は，運動しない人に比べて自分のダイエット計画を継続する傾向がある。(be apt to)

4. つぎの各問いに英語で答えなさい。

（1）What is the definition of BMI?

（2）Give five medical conditions associated with obesity.

（3）What are factors to cause obesity?

（4）What is the mainstay of treatment for obesity?

（5）What is the role of skeletal muscle in insulin pathway?

（6）What is your value of BMI? Are you in the healthy condition? If yes, how do you keep this situation? If not, how do you improve your body weight and BMI?

Chapter 15 Elderly Care

15.1 The Definition of Elderly Care

We live in a world that changes from moment to moment, a world in which we grow old, fall ill, and die. Since none of us can avoid birth, aging, sickness, and death, a time will probably come when we need to be cared for by others. Care is provided when someone can no longer independently carry out essential everyday activities like eating, bathing, dressing, etc. Care for the elderly is a major concern for all who live in an aging society.

Elderly care emphasizes the social and personal requirements of senior citizens who need some assistance with daily activities (activities of daily living; ADL) and health care (length of life; LOL). Furthermore, elderly desire and deserve to age with dignity (respect of life; ROL) and quality (quality of life; QOL). The broad term encompasses such services as assisted living, adult day care, long term care, hospice care, and Alzheimer's care. It can be provided at home, in the community, in assisted living or in nursing homes. It is an important distinction, in that the design of housing, services, activities, employee training and such should be truly customer-focused approach.

15.2 Nursing Care Needs for the Elderly

The care needs required by elder are summarized as below.

1. Foods: Appropriate meals for the elderly who may have lost their

---

Notes :
activities of daily living (ADL)「日常生活活動」, length of life (LOL)「生命の延長」
respect of life (ROL)「尊厳のある生活」, quality of Life (QOL)「生活の質」

dentures and have difficulty chewing are important. Also, the elder are at risk of developing malnutrition or gastrointestinal symptoms such as diarrhea and food poisoning.

2. Excretion: Temporary toilets in shelters are difficult for elder to use. As a result they may drink less water, which can lead to dehydration. In addition, having to walk a long distance to toilets and any differences in the levels of the toilet may increase the risk of falls. Support is necessary to avoid possible problems.

3. Decreased mobility: Elderly living in shelters suffer a decrease in activity caused by various mental and physical factors. After disasters, more elderly complain about pain in their back or knees, however they are often unable to receive medical treatment or rehabilitative therapy. These factors decrease their ability to remain active and result in an increased risk of their becoming bedridden. Therefore, it is important to maintain their daily activities and prevent them becoming bedridden which will affect their subsequent quality of life.

4. Deterioration of health condition: The elderly often suffer from deterioration in their overall health due to an insufficient intake of nutrition and water, mental and physical fatigue caused by the disaster, and the poor living environment of the shelter. It is necessary to evaluate the health of the elderly and provide support to prevent the aggravation of chronic conditions.

5. Mental health: It is difficult for the elderly to secure a living place by themselves within a shelter. While they repeatedly move within the shelter and endure a poor living environment, psychological stress sometimes manifests as physical symptoms. PTSD (post-traumatic stress disorder) sometime develops in the elderly without

Note :
PTSD (post-traumatic stress disorder)「外傷後ストレス障害」

being noticed and the elderly may suffer from continuous psychological disturbances such as a sense of helplessness and anxiety about their future without prospects for restoring their lives. Others physiological symptoms such as depressive disorders, anxiety disorder, obsessive compulsive disorders, and psychosomatic disease. Therefore, it is very important to assess the mental state of the elderly and attempt to maintain and improve their mental health.

6. Risk of developing delirium: In addition to mental and physical fatigue, an acute change in the living environment within the shelter may cause a transient brain dysfunction (such as mental agitation, unclear speech, sleep disorder and forgetfulness), the symptoms of which can be mistaken for dementia.

7. Exacerbation of dementia symptoms: Physical condition caused by the disasters and acute changes in the living environment can exacerbate symptoms of dementia and development of dementia in the elderly. Monitor physical functions of dementia include vital signs, dehydration, constipation, incontinence and pain. Assessment of cognitive function includes memory disorder, disorientation, and misjudgment etc. Assessment of behavioral disorder includes hallucination, delusion, aimless wandering, unclean behavior, and pica etc.

Furthermore, others factors are should be noticed for elderly care such as sanitary problems, oral hygiene, respiratory infections, isolation in terms of information, and problems surroundings transfer from the shelter.

Elderly care concentrates on helping individuals to function as

Notes:
depressive disorders「うつ病」, anxiety disorder「不安障害」
obsessive compulsive disorders「強迫神経症, 強迫性障害」
psychosomatic disease「心身症」

well as possible and it requires time and energy. Since no one can cope alone with all demands of care, other family members need to be understanding and cooperative and provide emotional support, besides the caregiver. Families are often equal beneficiaries of care interventions, because a brief respite for the family caregiver is important. When we realize that caring for the elderly is not someone else's problems and that we ourselves may eventually need care, we can approach caring for elder consideration and kindness.

Exercise

1. つぎの 1 〜 52 の語に対応する英単語または英熟語を本文から選び出して書き込み，また発音しなさい（動詞は原形を記入しなさい）。

	Japanese	English		Japanese	English
1	老齢化，老化		11	噛む	
2	強調する		12	栄養失調	
3	望む，希望する		13	胃腸（部）の	
4	値する		14	下痢	
5	尊厳		15	食中毒	
6	包含する		16	排泄	
7	ホスピス（末期患者のための病院）		17	脱水症状	
8	特質，特徴		18	災害，大惨事	
9	顧客中心の		19	リハビリ療法	
10	総義歯		20	寝たきり	

Note：
caregiver「介護者」

Unit E　Preventive Medicine and Social Consideration

	Japanese	English		Japanese	English
21	悪化		37	認知機能	
22	疲労		38	記憶障害	
23	悪化させること		39	方向感覚の喪失	
24	我慢する		40	幻覚	
25	示す		41	妄想	
26	不安		42	徘徊	
27	障害		43	異常行動	
28	期待		44	異食症	
29	精神錯乱		45	衛生の	
30	興奮		46	口腔衛生	
31	睡眠障害		47	呼吸器感染	
32	認知症		48	うまく処理する	
33	病勢などの悪化		49	協力的な	
34	生命徴候		50	受ける人	
35	便秘		51	一時的休止	
36	失禁		52	思いやり	

2. つぎの各文が本文の内容と一致するものには T(True)，一致しないものには F(False) を，文末の（　）に記入しなさい。

（1）Elderly care is a variety of services that includes medical and non-medical care to the elderly who have a chronic illness or disability. （　）

（2）Elderly care can be only provided at home. （　）

（3）It is important to maintain the elderly daily activities and prevent them becoming bedridden which will affect their subsequent quality of life. (　　)

（4）To take care about the mental health of caregivers are also important for elderly care. (　　)

（5）Elderly care is only the responsibility of the caregiver. (　　)

3. つぎの日本語の各文を（　　）の中の語を用いて英語の文にしなさい（必要があれば単語を適切な形に変換しなさい）。

（1）時々刻々移り変わる世の中に生きつつ，人は年老い，病み，死を迎える。(…change from moment to moment…)

（2）お年寄りの介護は，すべての人にとって高齢社会を生きるうえで大事な問題の一つである。(…a major concern)

（3）高齢者の健康評価と慢性症状の悪化を防ぐために，サポートを提供することが必要である。(…necessary to…. provide support to….)

（4）居住環境における大幅な変化は脳の機能不全を引き起こすかもしれない。(acute change…may cause…)

（5）老人介護には時間も手間も要することであり，一人の介護者ですべてをカバーすることはできないのである。(…require…. cope alone…)

4．つぎの各問いに英語で答えなさい。

（1）What is the brief definition of care?

（2）What are the three key factors for elderly care?

（3）Give four examples of nursing care needs which are required by elderly.

（4）What are the symptoms of cognitive functions on dementia?

（5）Would you like to live in nursing homes or live with your children when you are elderly? Why?

Chapter 16　Medical Bioethics

16.1　Bioethics

Bioethics is the compound Greece words from "bios" which represents life or something concerning life and "ethikos" which represents ethics thereof. Bioethics deals with ethical and value issues gained from life science. Life science is directly associated with life and nature science, including medicine, biology, genetics, medical care, and environment etc. Bioethics is one of applied ethics fields to treat about practical problems in life science with the principles of moral philosophy. It broadly comprises medical ethics, health care ethics, animal welfare, environmental ethics, and gene ethics etc.

16.1.1　The major four principles of Bioethics, plus one

(1) **The principle of respect for autonomy**　This is expressed in the language of rights, by recognizing the right of individual to make choices. Valuing the individual as one who makes self-defining choices upon which s/he then acts and for which s/he is accountable. In medical bioethics view, patients have rights to choice and decide what treatments of medical care, which they prefer to. Also, doctors have

---

Notes :
medical bioethics「医療生命倫理学」, applied ethics「応用倫理学」
practical problems「実際問題」, moral philosophy「道徳学, 倫理学」
medical ethics「医療倫理」, health care ethics「ヘルスケア倫理」
animal welfare「動物福祉」, environmental ethics「環境倫理」
gene ethics「遺伝子倫理」, the principle of respect for autonomy「自律尊重原理原則」

duty to respect patients' decisions and protect the patients who do not have autonomy ability. The derived principles in medical care are truthfulness, confidentiality, and informed consent.

(2) **The principle of non-maleficence (not harming)** We do not have duty to benefit human being but we have responsibility not to harm other people. In medical bioethics view, what are the medical indications, risks and benefits, and alternatives of the treatment being proposed by medical profession?

(3) **The principle of beneficence (doing good)** Besides doing well, we should prevent from harm and eliminate or remove harm. General speaking, people do not have perfect duty to benefit human being and this means "general beneficence." However, medical profession must conform to "the principle of beneficence" and this means "specific beneficence."

(4) **The principle of justice (resource allocation)** We should give every member in society and fair opportunities in life. It also means "fair, equitable, and appropriate treatment in light of what is due or owed to persons." In medical bioethics views, it includes broadly fields such as medical insurance plan and medical resources allocation.

(5) **Trustworthiness** It is valuing being able to be counted on to act with integrity, to be honest and truthful and to keep one's promises.

Notes :
informed consent「『インフォームドコンセント』患者の自己決定権，情報を与えられたうえでの同意」
the principle of non-maleficence「被害防止原則」，medical profession「医療専門家」
the principle of beneficence「善行原則」，the principle of justice「正義原則」
medical insurance plan「医療保険制度」

16.2 Period Division of Bioethics Issues

Medical sociologist, Dr. Fox, Renee, said there are three periods of Bioethics issues in America as below.

（1） **First period**　　From the end of 1960's to the early of 1970's, the key issue is human experimentation and the setting up the principle of "informed consent." Human experiments were noticed from Nuremberg Trials after the World War II in 1946. Nazi doctors did human experimentation on Jew and prisoner of war on concentration camp and it resulted in human subject dead or permanent disability. These Nazi doctors were trailed and than built up "Nuremberg Code-10 rules for Permissible Mideical Experiments" in 1947 to make sure the voluntary consent of the human subject.

（2） **Second period**　　From the end of 1970's to middle of 1980's, key issues are related to "life" and "death."

A. Beginning life-abortion and infanticide : This is the debate between rights of the woman and rights of fetus, questions of personhood, and sanctity of human life. Especially pertaining to abortion laws (women can decide to abortion or not within three months of fetus), advocacy groups divide into two opinions in the United Sates. One of them is in favor of legal prohibition of abortion described themselves as pro-life. One of them is against legal restrictions on abortion and describe as pro-choice. Both are used to indicate the central principles in arguments for and against abortion: "Is the fetus a human being with a fundamental right to *life*?" for pro-life advocates, and, for

Notes :
human experimentation「人体実験」, Nuremberg Trials「ニュルンベルク裁判」
infanticide「新生児安楽死。直訳すれば嬰児殺し」, pro-life「妊娠中絶反対」
pro-choice「妊娠中絶賛成」

those who are pro-choice, "Does woman have the right to *choose* whether or not to have an abortion?" Moreover, from the quality of woman's life of view, whether women have self-determination to consider about abortion enhance sanctity of life or not.

B. Continuing life-organ transplantation: From 1970's till now, both the sources (organs shortage) and method of obtaining the donor organs to transplant are major ethical issues to consider, as well as the concept of "distributive justice." The concept of distributive justice-how to fairly divide recourses-arises around organ transplantation because there are not enough organs available for every one who needs. Other issues also include: 1. Whether organ transplantation causes possible risk and dangers to organ donors or organ recipients. 2. How to get the agreement authority from organ donors who do not have ability such as brain dead patients. 3. Ethical debates are from using some potential non-traditional sources of organs (alternative organ sources) such as animal organs, artificial organs, stem cells, and aborted fetuses.

C. Toward the end of life: Euthanasia (from Greek: good-death) sometimes know as "mercy-killing or physician-assisted death." This is the proactive of terminating the life of a person in a painless or minimally painful way in order to stop suffering or other undesired conditions in life. This may be voluntary or involuntary, and carried out with or without a physician. For some people, the most important question about euthanasia is "Is it wrong to kill an innocent human being?" Deontologists believe we all need rules to live by, and everyone recognizes the power behind the rules "Do not kill." However, some people choose to break this rule in some circumstances. Teleologists believe there are occasions when "the end justifies the means."

Issues are raise by euthanasia are such as: 1. *Is killing the same as letting die?* On the other hand, what is the difference between acts and omissions? Should the law require us or doctor to act a certain way, or merely stop us from acting in certain ways? 2. *What would happen if we legalized euthanasia?* Some augur that there are many people suffering greatly who would benefit hugely if euthanasia were legalized. Some are worried about the misuse on the elderly people with disability or who are unwell. 3. *Do we have a right to die?* Some people claim human have "a right to live" so we have "a right to die." Other people say we have a right to dignity (death with dignity), and that euthanasia can provide a dignified, peaceful death rather than a prolonged period of lost dignity and great suffering. Other issues are related to the end of life such as hospice or terminal care. For example: From most of the experiences of hospice for the terminal cancer patients suggest "how to take care of their spiritual needed and support them" are much more important to consider to allow euthanasia or not.

(3) **Third period** From the middle of 1980's, key issue is medical economics. Medical economic issues are such as: A. Healthy insurance system: Illness can strike at anytime, and so there is the danger that an uninsured person might get really ill and not be able to afford medical treatment because of the expensive fees. In order to prevent this, there are different kinds of a compulsory insurance system in different countries. For examples, all people living in Japan must be covered by some form of insurance. There are two medical insurance systems in Japan: "Social Insurance System" for those working at a company or office; and "National Health Insurance System" for those uncovered by the Social Insurance System.

B. Medical care for the aged: The elderly health care system is

Notes :
death with dignity 「尊厳死」, hospice 「ホスピス」
terminal care 「末期医療」, medical economics 「医療経済」

aimed at improving health and promoting welfare for the elderly by municipalities' implementation of prevention, treatment and functional occupational therapy and other health care programs in comprehensive manners.

C. Commercialization of the human body and its use as resources: On the end of 20th century, there are three major innovative creations on biotechnology such as clone animal in 1997 in England, stem cell in 1998 in United State of America, and Human Genome Project in 2000. Others such as regeneration medicine, surrogacy, and human cloning are all of the novel biotechnology for medical resources. How to use all of these novel biotechnologies as resources and commercialization of human body are key issues to be concerned in the future.

16.3 Bioethics and Religious: Ethical Aspects of Death-"Euthanasia"

Religious ethics also has an influence upon both personal opinion and the greater debate over bioethics. Opinions of euthanasia may be one of the examples as a combination of beliefs on its morality, and beliefs on the responsibility, ethical scope, and proper extent of governmental authorities in public policy (see ELSI issue on last paragraph). There are different concepts on each religion.

16.3.1 Buddhism

In Buddhism, ethics are rooted in concerns related to virtue, karma, and liberation rather than the views of a divine being. The Buddha himself showed tolerance of suicide by monks in two cases. The Japanese Buddhist tradition includes many stories of suicide by monks,

Notes:
clone animal「クローン動物，クローン生物」, regeneration medicine「再生医療」
karma「《仏教》業」

and suicide was used as a political weapon by Buddhist monks during the Vietnam War. But these were monks, and that makes a difference. In Buddhism, the way life ends has a profound impact on the way the new life will begin. So a person's state of mind at the time of death is important-their thoughts should be selfless and enlightened, free of anger, hate or fear. This suggests that suicide (and so euthanasia) is only approved for people who have achieved enlightenment and that the rest of us should avoid it.

16.3.2 Christian

Christians are generally opposed to euthanasia and physician-assisted suicide, on the grounds that it invades God's territory of life and death and has other ethical problems. However, this position is not universal. There are only two mentions of suicide in the Old Testament: King Saul (I Samuel 31: 4 in Bible) and David's counselor, Ahitophel (II Samuel 17: 23 in Bible), both of which required the assistance of another person and are thus comparable to euthanasia. In the former case, a soldier takes Saul's life at his request, and King David has the soldier executed for murder. In the New Testament, there is one instance of suicide: that of Judas Iscariot, who feels remorse after betraying Jesus and hangs himself (Matthew 27: 3-5). The Bible does not comment on either of these instances, though it has been noted that none of the persons who commit suicide in the Bible are heroic or sympathetic figures.

16.3.3 Hinduism

Hindu views of euthanasia and physician-assisted suicide vary, but they are all rooted in concerns about karma, reincarnation, and ahim-

Notes:
reincarnation「霊魂の再生」, ahimsa「不殺生」

sa (non-violence). According to Hindu beliefs, if a person commits suicide, he neither goes to the hell nor the heaven, but remains in the earth consciousness as a bad spirit nor wanders aimlessly till he completes his actual and allotted life time. Thereafter he goes to hell and suffers more severely. In the end, he returns to the earth again to complete his previous karma and start from there once again. Suicide puts an individual's spiritual clock in reverse.

16.4 ELSI and Future Tasks of Bioethics

ELSI: Ethical, Legal, and Social Issues

　　The purpose of the development of science and technology (S&T) is to enhancement of quality of life (QOL). While the rapid development of S&T enrich our daily lives, there are also arising some issues associated to Ethical, Legal, and Social Issues (ELSI). The National Human Genome Research Institute's (NHGRI) Ethical, Legal, and Social Implication Research Program represents the world's largest ELSI program. It recognized that the information gained from mapping and sequencing the human genome would profound implications for individuals, families, and society. Although this information would have the potential to dramatically improve human health, they realized it would raise a number of complex ethical, legal and social issues. For instances: How should this genetic information be interpreted and used? Who should have access to it? How can we people be protected from that harm that might result from its importer disclosure or use?

Notes:
Ethical, Legal and Social Issues (ELSI)「倫理的・法的・社会的問題」
Ethical, Legal, and Social Implication 「倫理的・法的・社会的問題に密接な関係のあることがら」

Bioethical issues are serious concern for all of us living in an era of "life-Manipulation." This is the reason why the new "supra-interdisciplinary" study of "bioethics" deal with issues relating to all integrated aspects of life's beginning, ending and quality, compared to the too narrow segmentation and ramification trends of traditional academic disciplines dealing with human and life issues separately. Besides issues on the former part that we discussed, there are still much more issues such as gene testing and privacy, eugenics, human gene therapy that are to be concerned. There are not correct answers to tell you what is right or what is wrong, based on the concepts of bioethics. Simply speaking, bioethics is love of life and suggesting the concepts to make decisions when you meet the dilemmas.

Exercises

1. つぎの 1 ～ 38 の語に対応する英単語または英熟語を本文から選び出して書き込み，また発音しなさい（動詞は原形を記入しなさい）。

	Japanese	English		Japanese	English
1	自主性		9	誠実	
2	優先権		10	妊娠中絶	
3	誠実性		11	～に関係がある	
4	守秘義務		12	尊厳	
5	責任		13	支持	
6	従う		14	臓器移植	
7	配分		15	安楽死	
8	信頼性		16	配分	

Unit E Preventive Medicine and Social Consideration

	Japanese	English		Japanese	English
17	移植者		28	侵略する	
18	代わりに使える		29	優生学	
19	無罪の		30	見合う，類似の	
20	義務学者		31	履行する	
21	目的学者		32	売る	
22	怠慢		33	勇敢な	
23	義務的な，強制的な		34	同情的な	
24	総合的な		35	生命の質	
25	代理人の役目		36	深遠な	
26	修道僧		37	影響	
27	開けた		38	ジレンマ	

2．つぎの各文が本文の内容と一致するものにはT(True)，一致しないものにはF(False)を，文末の（　）に記入しなさい。

（1）Bioethics deals with ethical and value issues gained from medical science.（　）

（2）The simply meaning of "non-maleficence" is not harming.（　）

（3）Source of organ transplantation is key ethical issue to be concerned.（　）

（4）In Buddhism, ethics are rooted in concerns related to virtue, karma, and liberation rather than the views of a divine being.（　）

（5）There are correct answers to tell you what is right or what is wrong, based on the concepts of bioethics.（　）

3．つぎの日本語の各文を（　　）の中の語を用いて英語の文にしなさい（必要があれば単語を適切な形に変換しなさい）。

（1）医師には，患者の決定を尊敬するとともに，自主的な能力をもっていない患者を保護する義務がある。(duty, respect, protect, autonomy ability)

（2）尊厳死とは，生命のあり方において苦痛や他の望まれない状況をできるだけ避ける手段として，苦痛を最低限に抑えてその生命を終焉させる考え方と行為である。(terminate, undesired, suffer, pain)

（3）医療費は高価であり，医療保険がないと多大な出費が患者の負担となる。そして，病気は予測できずに突然起こる。(strike, uninsured person, afford, medical treatment)

（4）宗教倫理学は，生命倫理のうえで個人的な見解と大きな論争の両方から影響を受ける。(have an influence, debate)

4．つぎの各問いに英語で答えなさい。
（1）What is bioethics? Explain this briefly.

(2) What are the major principles of Bioethics?

(3) What are the three periods of Bioethics, based on the theory of Dr. Fox, Renee?

(4) What is ELSI? Explain this briefly.

(5) How do you think about euthanasia? Do you agree about this?

References

Chapter 1
1) 日本薬剤師会編：第 11 改訂　調剤指針（増補版），添付文書中の「警告」，「禁忌」の確認，pp.54 〜 56，薬事日報社（December 2002）
2) くすりのカルテ研究会編，荒井なおみ，ほか著：薬歴管理と服薬指導，薬歴管理サブノート，pp.81 〜 100，南山堂（April 2003）
3) 堀岡正義：調剤学総論 改訂 8 版，TDM に必要な薬物動態理論の基礎知識；第 8 章　血中薬物濃度モニタリング（TDM）概論，pp.188 〜 193，薬物相互作用・併用禁忌；第 9 章　配合と併用，pp.197 〜 242，南山堂（April 2006）
4) くすりの絵文字（ピクトグラム）英語版，くすりの情報ステーション（ネット版），http://www.rad-ar.or.jp/english/index.html（2008 年 3 月現在）

Chapter 2
1) 日本薬学会編：SBO 50，第 IV 部，薬学への招待，第 16 章 薬について，ヒューマニズム・薬学入門，pp.220 〜 227，東京化学同人（April 2005）
2) 日本薬学会編：医薬品の研究開発プロセス，高校生および大学初年度生のための薬学紹介パワーポイント教材，日本薬学会（May 2006）
3) 薬害資料館（ネット版），http://www.mi-net.org/yakugai/（2006 年 4 月現在）

Chapter 3
1) 鷲谷いづみ，矢原徹一：保全生態学入門，文一総合出版（1996）
2) 樋口広芳編：保全生物学，東京大学出版会（1996）
3) T. Watanabe and A. Takano : The Role of Botanical Gardens on International Cooperation in the Field of Plant Genetic Resources 36, pp.132 〜 135 (2002)
4) T. Watanabe and A. Takano : Survey of wildflowers in Amazon(2), Utilization of Brazilian medicinal plants lower Amazon River. Aroma Research, (Journal of Aroma Science and Technology), 123(4), pp.84 〜 92 (2002)
5) 今西二郎，二本柳賢司編：別冊医学のあゆみ「世界の伝統医学」，医歯薬出版（1997）

Chapter 4
1) http://www.igm.hokudai.ac.jp/crg/zoonosis/
2) http://www.primate.or.jp/PF/yamanouchi/index.html
3) http://www.bayer-pet.jp/pet/zoonosis/index.html
4) http://www.shiga-med.ac.jp/~hqanimal/

Chapter 7
1) A. Griffith, et al. : Modern Genetic Analysis 2nd edition, Chapter 11. Chromosome mutation, Frfeeman and Co., NY. (2002)
2) L. H. Hartwell, et al. : Genetics, Chapter 13. Chromosome rearrangements and Changes in Chromosome Number Reshape Eukaryotic Genomes. McGraw Hill, Boston (2004)
3) C. P. Swanson, et al. : Cytogenetics. Prentice Hall, Englewood Cliffs, NJ, USA (1981)

Chapter 8
1) http://www.asgt.org/
2) http://www.nature.com/gt/index.html
3) L. H. Hartwell, et al. : Genetics - From Genes to Genomes-. 2nd edition, Page 29, 218, 361 and 380. ISBN:0-07-291930-2, McGrawHill, London (2004)
4) K. Massimini : Genetic Disorders Sourcebook. 2nd edition, Omnigraphics Inc. NY. ISBN:978-078080241-4 (2001)

Chapter 9
1) I. L. Weissman : Stem cells - Units of Development, Units of Regeneration and Units in Evolution-. Cell, 100, pp.157 ～ 168 (2000)
2) http://stemcells.nih.gov/info/basics/

Chapter 10
1) C. J. Koh and A. Atala : Therapeutic cloning applications for organ transplantation. Transplant immunology 12, pp.193 ～ 201 (2004)
2) http://www.fda.gov/cber/xap/xap.htm
3) http://www.cdc.gov/ncidod/eid/vol2no1/michler.htm

Chapter 11
1) M. A. Horton and A. Khan : Medical nanotechnology in the UK ; a perspective from the London Centre for Nanotechnology, Nanomedicine: Nanotechnology, Biology and Medicine 2: pp.42 ～ 48 (2006)
2) http://nihroadmap.nih.gov/nanomedicine/
3) http://cordis.europa.eu/nanotechnology/nanomedicine.htm

Chapter 12
1) M. Asada, K. F. MacDroman, H. Ishiguro and Y. Kuniyoshi : Cognitive development robotics as a new paradigm for the designing humanoid robots. Robotics and Autonomous Systems 37, pp.185 ～ 193 (2001)
2) http://ci.nii.ac.jp/naid/110000136723/en/

3) http://ci.nii.ac.jp/naid/110001130405/en/

Chapter 13
1) I. Wickelgren : A vision for blind. Science 312, pp.1124 〜 1126 (2006)
2) http://www.wicab.com/

Chapter 14
1) C. P. Fenster, et al. : Obesity, aerobic exercise, and vascular disease: the role of oxidant stress. Obesity Research 10 (9), pp. 964 〜 968 (2002)
2) P. G. Kopelman : Obesity as a medical problem. Nature 404, pp. 635 〜 643 (2000)
3) L. S. Pescatello, et al. : The muscle strength and size response to upper arm, unilateral resistance training among adults who are overweight and obese. Journal of Strength and Conditioning Research 21(2), pp. 307 〜 313 (2007)

Chapter 15
1) 播本高志編著：絵でわかる！疲れない，疲れさせない介護，PHP研究所（2007）
2) 住居広士，ほか編：見てよくわかる，リハビリテーション介護技術（新訂版），一橋出版（2007）
3) The 21st Century Center of Excellence Program, Nursing care provider guidance for elderly in shelters following disasters (First edition), Center of Disaster of Excellence Program, University of Hyogo (2005)

Chapter 16
1) 加藤尚武，飯田亘之編，H.T. エンゲルハート，H. ヨナス，ほか著：バイオエシックスの基礎—欧米の「生命倫理」論，東海大学出版会（1998）
2) 今井道夫，香川知晶編：バイオエシックス入門—生命倫理入門（第2版），東信堂（1996）
3) 加藤尚武，加茂直樹編：生命倫理学を学ぶ人のために，世界思想社（1998）
4) 市野川容孝編：生命倫理とは何か，平凡社（2002）
5) http://www.genome.gov
6) http://www.rsrevision.com/Alevel/ethics/euthanasia/index.htm

Answers to Exercises

Chapter 1
Exercises 1
1. tannin, 2. catechin, 3. anemia, 4. attenuate, 5. palpitation, 6. nausea,
7. mitigate, 8. alleviate, 9. nasal, 10. laxatives, 11. citrus, 12. flavonoid,
13. naringenin, 14. xenobiotics, 15. antagonist, 16. sedative drug,
17. antipyretic drug, 18. analgesic drug, 19. cephem antibiotics,
20. deterrent, 21. concomitant, 22. sensation, 23. tranquilizer,
24. esophagus, 25. ulcer, 26. adverse reactions, 27. pharmacochemical,
28. expiration date, 29. ophthalmic, 30. take it before a meal,
31. take it between meals, 32. take it after a meal, 33. compliance,
34. appetite, 35. hypoglycemia, 36. asthma, 37. irrespective of,
38. hypnotic drugs, 39. nocturnal, 40. anti-ulcerative drugs,
41. antiemetic drugs, 42. suppository, 43. anus, 44. attainable

Exercises 2
(1) F, (2) F, (3) T, (4) F, (5) T, (6) F

Exercises 3
(1) Because it becomes difficult for drugs to solve in the stomach when the drugs are taken without water, it becomes slow-acting. In addition, might it stick to the gullet of the mouth and causes inflammation. The purpose of the pharmacist's saying, "Please drink by one glass of water" is to be often effective because it is not only to drink easily.

(2) Do not take an iron content alone to improve anemia. It leads to the production capacity decrease of the red blood cell if the protein is not enough to be taken. Especially, people will refrain from meat and the fish with a lot of proteins when dieting, the hem iron with a good iron absorption causes anemia running short and doubly, too.

(3) The drugs prescribed by the doctor are called, "Ethical pharmaceutical", and the effect is large because what suitable for the person's condition is prescribed, and the side effect is also strong. On the other hand, drugs that we usually buy in the drugstore etc. are called, "Non-prescription pharmaceutical", and the side effect has decreased comparatively mildly as for the action, too. These mean "Store-based sales" as an OTC drug.

(4) The elements having both strengthens the effect of drugs in the smoke of cigarette and shortens the duration of the effect are contained. Therefore, stopping smoking during the treatment period and the period before and after that is important.

(5) "Medical supplies reasonable advertisement standard" is installed in the target drug for the drug legislation, and an easy advertisement is not admitted. However, PR release never admitted in the drug legislation such as 'In a moment effect' or 'I have recovered, too' revolts to the street as shown in the public.

Exercises 4

(1) One reason for tabooing taking drugs with tea is not to be absorbed in the intestinal tract because tannin contained in tea binds with iron.

(2) No, because it becomes difficult for drugs to solve in the stomach without water, and slow-acting. Also it might stick to the gullet of the mouth and causes inflammation.

(3) No, because even unopened drugs kept in a proper place under proper conditions undergo changes in ingredient quality little by little everyday, and drugs may lose their efficacy or even become harmful.

(4) As an inflammation is caused by the friction of the skin when patient strongly rubs ointment, I recommend applying small quantity of ointment into several times on a hand.

(5) No, in fact calcium and protein contained in milk binds with the ingredient and attenuates the effectiveness of the drugs.

(6) Because the drug remains in the stomach or sticks to the wall of stomach when the drug is taken while having slept, the drug doesn't melt easily. Therefore, you had better up to take.

Chapter 2
Exercises 1

1. drug, 2. supreme, 3. promoting the health, 4. reasonability, 5. safety,
6. absorption, 7. distribution, 8. metabolism, 9. excretion, 10. premature,
11. criteria, 12. escalate, 13. streamline, 14. renovation, 15. new drug,

16. forecasted, 17. marketability, 18. profitability, 19. clinical, 20. possibility,
21. patent application, 22. intellectual property, 23. analytical chemistry,
24. quality control, 25. animal experiment, 26. acute toxicity,
27. subacute toxicity, 28. chronic toxicity, 29. tentatively,
30. ADRs(side effect), 31. penicillin shock, 32. thalidomide, 33. antibiotic,
34. infection

Exercises 2

(1) F, (2) T, (3) T, (4) F, (5) F, (6) T

Exercises 3

(1) The modern life for people has been improved with the chemical substances. A lot of things such as a medicine, cosmetics, a food additive, a utensil, an industrial chemistry products, and architectural materials are found in the world as a chemical substance.

(2) The viruses are different for influenza and usual cold. A usual cold is caused by influenza because of adenovirus, rhinovirus and the bacillus, etc.

(3) The total cost is suppressed to a half price of the new medicine with averaging though the generic medicine is the same as both element and effect as new medicine because a high development cost reduction and shortening at the development period are more possible than the new medicine. Therefore, the load of charge for the medicine of patient is able not only to be reduced but also to contribute to medical-expenses reduction in our country.

(4) At least, 30 % of the inpatient receives the treatments with antibiotic one or any more, and the million kinds of infectious disease related to life and death are treated in present.

(5) The life of Japanese became rich, and epidemics such as dysentery, cholera, and tuberculosis were not the fatal diseases though the treatment method to be established with the advancement of public health and the enhancements of health and medical treatment. However, treatment is difficult and the illness which follows chronic progress also still exists. Such diseases are called an intractable disease.

Exercises 4

(1) No, it isn't. For example about Penicillin, it was drastically effective for infections. However, in 1956, a patient developed allergy reaction with severe shock called anaphylactic shock after receiving an injection of penicillin. If the antibiotic is used for a long time, the resistant bacteria will appear and an effect will be lost. Moreover, any antibiotic has side effects, so that means not to an omnipotent medicine.

(2) What did not being a new drug, these will be reborn to agricultural chemicals etc. instead of a new medicine.

(3) The cold remedies such as aminopyrine or sulpyrin are contained. These chemical substances caused to deaths in Japan.

(4) Every medicine will cast a big shadow over society, such as a lawsuit on adverse drug reactions by the side-effects damage of a medicine, after approval of new medicines production. As part of the improvement of the system for compensating victims of drug disaster, various frameworks have been enforced for checking the processes to manufacturing, approval and launch.

(5) It need to have side-effects information sufficiently from the doctor or the pharmacist about the prescription medicine and OTC drugs. And it is important that patient also arranges the information about medicine in everyday life.

(6) The technology doesn't develop without basic research. In the medicinal world, we surely thinks about new technologies such as a cause elucidation about disease, a diagnostic and a screening method, it can be proceed to be rich the life of people will be rich. However, it cannot be lead the peace to people without nuclear peaceful use.

Chapter 3
Exercises 1

1. profit distribution, 2. convention on biological diversity (CBD),
3. ecological, 4. national inventory, 5. higher plant,
6. sustainable development, 7. National Cancer Institute (NCI),
8. rheumatoid arthritis, 9. antibody, 10. artificial organ, 11. rejection,
12. plant biotechnology, 13. animal protection, 14. vaccine,
15. blood product, 16. immunity fortifier,
17. biological decomposition plastic, 18. industrial use enzyme, 19. rejection

Answers to Exercises

Exercises 2
(1) T, (2) F, (3) T, (4) F, (5) T, (6) F

Exercises 3
(1) The United States thought that it was necessary to give priority to the method of not the excessive handling of the plant inheritance resource but use according to the purpose, and to secure a free access of the resource enough.

(2) When biotechnology is divided roughly, it is classified into animal cell culture system biotechnology, microorganism system biotechnology, and plant system biotechnology. Recently, the risk of the bacillus infection of the cow disease etc. and the serum production using the animal are put in question as for animal cell culture system biotechnology of the main current because of an ethical side of protection etc.

(3) There are a lot of advantages that the material production process such as the medicines utilized plant biotechnology is an environmental harmony type process where the negative environmental impact is few, and the investment and the running cost to the production facility etc. are suppressed to low.

(4) The model project of local based type considered the environment issues has been developed by preserving the environment and promoting industrialization at the same time, though it seems to conflict in the Himalayan mountain's region.

(5) The researchers who know the value of anxiety nature for exhaustion of plant resources are tackling the study of sterile multiplication by plant biotechnology. However, by the time while it demonstrates the result, further more time and expense will be required.

Exercises 4
(1) These projects such as having the policies without exploitation from the natures, will be very helpful to local people. And it is also another purpose to establish the way of cash earnings in the farmer who advances plant industrialization.

(2) It means that raw materials of medicine are not enough. About the plant materials which will be much quantity used as raw materials of the medicine, we are for protecting these resources the research on establishment and the plant propagation using plant cultivation techniques will surely be continued constantly.

(3) The biological diversity is also the guideline to healthy the earth environment including a human being. However, the real worth to the biological diversity through CBD is not acknowledged in the developing countries.

(4) For example about anticancer drug, there are the alkaloid Taxol isolated from yew tree as *Taxus brevifolia* Hort. ex Gord and Yunnan yew tree as *Taxus yunnanensis*.

(5) Alkaloid Camptothecine was isolated from happy tree (Chinese : Xi Shu) having the scientific name of *Camptotheca acuminata*.

(6) A threshold is only made high to the company which enters into the plant industrial field, and industrialization does not progress, the way of the cash earnings of a spot will be shut.

Chapter 4
Exercises 1
1. pathogen, 2. pest, 3. infect, 4. zoonosis, 5. bit, 6. injury, 7. gut, 8. liver,
9. veterinarian, 10. rabies, 11. toxocarosis, 12. toxoplasmosis, 13. acute,
14. encephalitis, 15. inflammation, 16. brain, 17. mammalian, 18. avian,
19. inapparent infection, 20. protozoa, 21. embryo, 22. fetus, 23. abortion,
24. athlete foot, 25. dermatophytosis, 26. endemic, 27. echinococcosis,
28. echinocuccus, 29. vector, 30. mediate, 31. predator, 32. infest,
33. prevention, 34. ourbreak, 35. host, 36. haemorrhagic,
37. epidemiological, 38. incidence, 39. specificity, 40. poultry, 41. excrement,
42. inhale, 43. involuntary, 44. hygiene, 45. sanitation, 46. creature

Exercises 2
(1) T, (2) F, (3) F, (4) T, (5) F

Exercises 3
(1) Athlete foot is one of dermatophytoses, and it is the zoonosis which cause mutual infection among humans and animals.

(2) The outbreaks of various infectious diseases become global concerns in the past several decades.

(3) SARS was not spread by masked palm civet cat and roccoons, The bat species are regarded as the natural hosts.

(4) Marburg virus causes haemorrhagic fever, and infected victims could face a high probability of death. This virus is also mediated by bat as the natural host.

(5) Toxosoplasmosis is caused by protozoo species. Generally speaking it is inapparent infection and there is no major concern, however, when the embryo is infected, it could cause abortion of the fetus or substantial damage to the baby after the birth.

Exercises 4

(1) Those pathogens and pests which can commonly infect human and animals.

(2) They could be natural hosts for serious pathogenic agents such as viruses.

(3) It is better to avoid direct exposures to wild animals as they could carry human infectious pathogens or pests. Especially injury by bites should be treated immediately.

(4) It is proteinaceous infectious particle, and this causes Creutzfeldt-Jakob disease.

(5) There are many examples such as rabies, SARS, ebola virus, toxocarosis and athlete foot.

Chapter 5
Exercises 1

1. parasite, 2.malaria, 3.symptom, 4. chills, 5.diarrhea, 6. estimated,
7. infection, 8. annually, 9. vaccine, 10. formidable, 11. intense,
12. systematic, 13. candidate, 14. sporozoite, 15. circulation,
16. hepatocyte, 17. parasitized, 18. erythrocyte, 19. complicated,
20. complexity, 21. parasite, 22. feasibility,
23. *Plasmodium falciparum* parasites, 24. sterile, 25. immunity,
26. immunization, 27. radiation, 28. attenuated, 29. manifestation,
30. efficacious, 31. warrant, 32. consortium, 33. anticipated, 34. facilitate,
35. intervention, 36. diagnostics, 37. putative, 38. expressed sequence tag,
39. bioinformatics, 40. corresponding to, 41. exploited, 42. identification,
43. prioritization, 44. epitope

Exercises 2
(1) T, (2) T, (3) F, (4) F, (5) T

Exercises 3
(1) Recent analyses show that about 1.5 ~ 3 million malaria-infected deaths occurred annually.
(2) Despite a relatively intense research effort conducted since the 1960s, few humans have been protected from malaria infection.
(3) The first model to design a malaria vaccine is to induce sterile immunity in humans by immunization with radiation-attenuated sporozoites.
(4) The second model to design a malaria vaccine is to induce erythrocytic stage immunity to prevent disease of naturally acquired immunity.
(5) The genomic sequence data provide a set of bioinformatics corresponding to potential malaria target antigens.

Exercises 4
(1) A bite from a mosquito infected with certain parasites may cause malaria.
(2) Because developing a vaccine against malaria is complicated by the complexity of parasite as well as the complexity of the host's response to the parasite.
(3) Two models have been suggested to develop a malaria vaccine.
(4) The two models provided merits to prevent all clinical manifestations and prevent death and severe disease of naturally acquired immunity.
(5) An international consortium of genome scientists and funding agencies was formed to sequence the genome of malaria in 1996.

Chapter 6
Exercises 1
1. dementia, 2. dementious, 3. ailment, 4. senile, 5. cerebrovascular,
6. vascular disorder, 7. atherosclerosis, 8. hypertension,
9. schemic heart disease, 10. hyperlipidemia, 11. diabetic, 12. degradation,
13. neuron, 14. rigidity, 15. resting tremor, 16. postural instability,
17. akinesia, 18. bradykinesia, 19. autonomic nervous system,
20. depression, 21. neuro-physiological, 22. heritable, 23. gene,
24. cognitive impairment, 25. disorientation, 26. spatial sense,

27. autosomal chromosome, 28. pathological, 29. atrophy, 30. senile plaque,
31. cerebral cortex, 32. deposition, 33. cerebrum, 34. epidemiological,
35. occurrence, 36. epidemiological, 37. deter, 38. persecution mania,
39. hallucination, 40. stakeholder, 41. care-taker, 42. abusive,
43. unintentional loitering, 44. filty, 45. vulnerable, 46. ancestral

Exercises 2

(1) T, (2) T, (3) F, (4) T, (5) T

Exercises 3

(1) This chapter focuses on Alzheimer's disease, while brief statements are made generally on dementious disorders.

(2) Vascular ailments are often originated from the lifestyle customs.

(3) Anybody can have a risk to Parkinson Disease with the progress of aging.

(4) AD progresses gradually and serious levels of AD could cause troubles in eating, changing cloths and communications, which requires the assistance of care-takers.

(5) The patients with dimentious disorders would cause persecution mania and/or hallucination with its disease progress.

Exercises 4

(1) There are a lot of patience and consideration with the vulnerable people. Think that if you were to be such a condition.

(2) One can recommend reduce unhealthy life behaviors such as overeating meats, lack of appropriate exercises and day to day consideration on own life.

(3) The progress of the AD could be deterred by using medicaments. Example would be cholinesterase inhibitors such as donepezil hydrochloride.

(4) The general appearance symptoms are: rigidity, resting tremor, postural instability, akinesia, and bradykinesia, and also often observation are seen such on the disorders in autonomic nervous system, depression and dementia.

(5) The biological research is one to pursue, oriented to practices. However, ethics, legal and social systems should be sophisticated to accommodate such patients without burden of direct commitment of families.

Chapter 7
Exercises 1
1. chromosome, 2. trisomics, 3. hereditary/heredity, 4. genetic/genetics,
5. aneuploid/aneuploidy, 6. deletion, 7. duplication, 8. inversion,
9. translocation, 10. aberration, 11. polyploidy, 12. polyploidization,
13. monosomy, 14. trisomy, 15. monosomics, 16. nullisomics, 17. cytogenetics,
18. fatal, 19. gametic/gamete, 20. embryonic/embryo, 21. nondisjunction,
22. mitosis, 23. meiosis, 24. chemical mutagen, 25. malnutrition,
26. interference, 27. utero (uterus), 28. autosome, 29. rudimentary ovary,
30. gonadal streak, 31. sterile, 32. constriction, 33. aorta, 34. deformity,
35. testicular insufficiency, 36. tetrasomy, 37. pentasomy, 38. osteoporosis,
39. retardant, 40. reproduce, 41. fertile, 42. imbalance, 43. vulnerable

Exercises 2
(1) F, (2) F, (3) T, (4) F, (5) T

Exercises 3
(1) Chromosomal abnormalities can be observed in any higher organisms.
(2) Genetic disorders associate with diverse genetic factors and chromosomal aberrations are included as a major category.
(3) Polyploidy and aneuploidy can be observed generally in Plant kingdom. Polyploids are common occurrence at angiosperms in nature.
(4) Chromosomal abnormalities are fatal at gametic or embryonic stages in mammalians.
(5) Chromosomal nondisjunction can happen by chance.

Exercises 4
(1) It increases the frequency by interference with microtubules polymerization action by more exposures to chemical mutagens, radiation, extraordinary temperatures for organisms.
(2) See the main text.
(3) Persons with the syndrome have testicular insufficiency and are lanky build, sterile, more chance to osteoporosis, and some mentally retardant with slightly feminized physical appearance including breast development.
(4) The trisomy at Chromosome 21 is the cause on the Down syndrome.
(5) No it could happen at any family.

Chapter 8
Exercises 1
1. genome, 2. occurrence, 3. immunological dysfunction, 4. alteration,
5. locus, 6. mutation, 7. deletion, 8. substitution, 9. insertion,
10. nucleic acid, 11. sickle cell anemia, 12. hemoglobin, 13. molecule,
14. codominant, 15. restriction enzyme, 16. allele, 17. blood clotting,
18. hemophilia, 19. bleed, 20. recessive, 21. hypophosphatemia,
22. dominant, 23. rickets, 24. cystic fibrosis, 25. probability, 26. mucus,
27. failure, 28. fatal, 29. genetic engineering, 30. transgenic, 31. somatic,
32. administer, 33. ethics, 34. prejudice, 35. insurance, 36. employment,
37. vulnerable

Exercises 2
(1) F, (2) F, (3) F, (4) T, (5) F

Exercises 3
(1) Huntington's disease is a fatal, autosomal-dominant neurological illness causing involuntary movements, severe emotional disturbance and cognitive decline.
(2) Hemophilia is incompletion or failing of blood clotting and it is controlled by recessive sex-linked inheritance on X chromosome.
(3) Gene therapy is the genetic engineering method to alter the genetic nature by inserting a gene fragment into human genome for changing the function of the target disease-causing gene(s) to reduce or eliminate the disease.
(4) Ethical considerations should be made on handling the genetic information of individuals as described in the last chapter of this book.
(5) The difference between normal and disease-causing alleles, can be detected by the combination of molecular biology approaches.

Exercises 4
(1) No one can deny the possibility of having a genetic disorder on oneself.
(2) Cytic fibrosis, hypophosphatemia caused disorders and hemophilia are all genetic diseases. However, the modern medical sciences have been alleviating the problems by various approaches with promoting research on the causes and mechanisms and genetics of the illness.
(3) The cause of the genetic disease, could be a minor alteration of a locus,

by a mutation based on deletion, substitution and/or insertion of nucleic acids or DNA.
(4) Huntington's disease is caused by a dominant allele on Chromosome 4.
(5) Individual genetic information could be used for various social activities, but the deep consideration must be made on the ethical aspects.

Chapter 9
Exercises 1
1. regeneration, 2. evolution, 3. capable, 4. self-renewal, 5. multilineage,
6. differentiation, 7. subset, 8. retain, 9. ultimately, 10. progeny,
11. irreversible, 12. maturation, 13. characterized, 14. postconception,
15. yolk sac 16. vasculature, 17. presumably, 18. migration,
19. microenvironment, 20. successive, 21. mobilization, 22. transplantation,
23. autoimmunity, 24. lethal dose, 25. irradiation, 26. chemotherapy,
27. mammalian, 28. somatic tissues, 29. primitive

Exercises 2
(1) F, (2) T, (3) T, (4) T, (5) F

Exercises 3
(1) Stem cells are not only units of biological organization, responsible for the development and the regeneration of tissue and organ systems, but also are units in evolution by natural selection.
(2) Each stage of differentiation involves functionally irreversible maturation steps.
(3) Hematopoietic stem cells are probably the best characterized stem cell population.
(4) Understanding the biology of HSCs has led to a number of medical advances in cancer therapy, trnaplantation, and autoimmunity.
(5) Stem cells other than HSCs in mammalian somatic tissue are found capable of generating somatic systems.

Exercises 4
(1) The two main properties of stem cells are self-renewal and multilineage differentiation.
(2) Short-term set of stem cells differentiate into multipotent progenitors

which then differentiate into oligolinage progenitors and finally give rise to differentiated progeny.

(3) Hematopoiesis occurs in the yolk sac blood island, and the yolk sac vasulature connects via the umbilical vein to the fetal liver.

(4) The changes in expression of cell surface adhesion molecules may control the movement of HSC from embryonic to fetal liver.

(5) Stem cells derived from primitive endoderm, including gut, liver and pancreas are candidates for the application of organ regeneration.

Chapter 10
Exercises 1
1. restore, 2. perform, 3. transplant, 4. allogeneic, 5. genetically, 6. dissimilar,
7. unrelated, 8. recipient, 9. overcome, 10. immunologic, 11. barrier,
12. revolutionary, 13. era, 14. therapy, 15. injured, 16. shortage,
17. availability, 18. treatment, 19. spawn, 20. alternative, 21. embryo,
22. explanted, 23. stem cell, 24. identical, 25. replacement, 26. ban,
27. clinically, 28. strategy, 29. acelullar, 30. matrices, 31. cellular,
32. component, 33. mechanical, 34. manipulation, 35. collagen-rich,
36 .degrade, 37.ingrowing, 38. dissociate, 39. cultured, 40. expansion,
41. adequate, 42. seeded, 43. synthesize, 44. replicate, 45. biomaterial,
46. delivery, 47. bioactive,

Exercises 2
(1) F, (2) F, (3) F, (4) T, (5) T

Exercises 3
(1) Organ transplantation is one of the first methods to restore from and function in modern medicine.

(2) Therapeutic cloning is used to generate early stage embryos that are explanted in culture to produce embryonic stem cells lines.

(3) Autologous stem cells have the potential to become almost any type of cell in the adult body.

(4) Most current strategy for tissue/organ replacement is tissue engineering.

(5) A small piece of donor tissue or cloned tissue is dissociated into individual cells which are then cultured in vitro for sufficient expansion of adequate number.

Exercises 4

(1) Allogeneic organ transplantation is a transplantation in which an organ from a genetically dissimilar donor into an unrelated recipient.

(2) Because a severe shortage of donor organs limits the availability of this treatment.

(3) Therapeutic cloning and tissue engineering are developed to replace organ transplantation.

(4) Acellular tissue matrices are prepared by removing cellular components from tissues via mechanical and chemical manipulation to produce collagen-rich matrices.

(5) The expand cells are seeded onto a scaffold synthesized with appropriate biomaterials which can replicate the biologic and mechanical function of native ECM so as to form a three-dimensional space for the cells to form into new tissues with appropriate structure and function.

Chapter 11
Exercises 1

1. nanotechnology, 2. atom, 3. molecule, 4. novel, 5. nanoscale, 6. billionth,
7. broadly, 8. bottom-up, 9. top-down, 10. physically, 11. minute, 12. probe,
13. location, 14. intricately, 15. carve, 16. heavy metal, 17. hipe, 18. coerce,
19. bridge, 20. capability, 21. diverse, 22. nanotube, 23. superconductor,
24. organic, 25. carbon, 26. silicon, 27. organic material, 28. deliverables,
29. real-space, 30. label-free, 31. diagnostics, 32. tracer, 33. pharmaceutical,
34. petrochemical, 35. biocompatible, 36. tool kit, 37. misfolded, 38. grasp,
39. unravel, 40. refold, 41. fundamental, 42. inhibit, 43. free up

Exercises 2

(1) T, (2) T, (3) F, (4) F, (5) T

Exercises 3

(1) It is possible to push atoms into a desired location using atomically fine force microscope tips.

(2) At present, the novel nanotechnology bridges the biological and nonbiological worlds.

(3) Techniques covering areas such as superconductors and carbon nanostructures have been built.

(4) Nanotechnology has extended to aspect of health care, especially the low-cost diagnostics and novel drug delivery systems.

(5) Researching the cause of diseases lies in a greater understanding of the structure an function of proteins.

Exercises 4

(1) Nanotechnology involves the precise manipulation and control of atoms and molecules to create novel materials with properties controlled at the nanoscale.

(2) The bottom-up approach involves manipulating small numbers of atoms or molecules into structures by minute probes, while the top-down approach involves growing atoms and molecules and moving them to a desired location or structures.

(3) The aspect of health care, especially the low-cost diagnostics and novel drug delivery system.

(4) Examples of the deliverables in the area of nanomedicines are: real-space images of biomolecules, label-free rapid protein and DNA diagnostics, individually tailed drugs and selective delivery systems, tracers for pharmaceutical, biocompatible scaffolds for tissue engineering, and mobile network-based health care.

(5) Alzheimer's disease is linked to misfolded proteins. Nanotechnology can watch proteins unravel and refold in their natural environments.

Chapter 12
Exercises 1

1. heroines, 2. motivated, 3. communicate, 4. physical, 5. entity, 6. explicitly,
7. implement, 8. physics, 9. interaction, 10. cognition, 11. interface,
12. fundamental, 13. mankind, 14. synthetic, 15. constructive, 16. potential,
17. diagnosis, 18. reimplementation, 19. iterate, 20, refinement,
21. significantly, 22. embed, 23. dynamics, 24. cooperative, 25. competitive,
26. promising

Exercises 2

(1) F, (2) F, (3) T, (4) T, (5) F

Exercises 3
(1) Robot heroes in science fiction movies and cartoons like Star Wars do not exit in real world.
(2) The robots in movies, unlike special purpose machines, are able to communicate with us.
(3) Recent progress promoted a new area called developmental cognitive neuroscience.
(4) The cycle of fault diagnosis and reimplementation may iterate many times in order to refine the model.
(5) This process of refinement is expected to result in a useful model of human interaction.

Exercises 4
(1) CDR was started to aim to understand the cognitive developmental processes that an intelligent root would require and how to realize them in a physical entity.
(2) The difference is that existing approaches often explicitly implement a control structure in the robot's brain that was derived from a designer's understanding of the robot's physics, while the CDR structures reflects the robot's own process of understanding through interactions with the environment.
(3) DCN emerges at the interface between cognitive neuroscience and development.
　The former concerns the relation between the mind and the body, and the latter concerns the origin of organized biological structure such as the structure of adult human brain.
(4) The design principle of CDR is a self-developing structure which is embedded inside the robot's brain, and an outside environment is set up so that the robot embedded structure can learn and develop from the environment and gradually adapt itself to more complex tasks in more dynamic situations.
(5) The intelligent robot will learn the response to the other active agents such as cooperative, competitive or both responses.

Chapter 13
Exercises 1
1. advanced, 2. experimental, 3. device, 4. crude, 5. inadequate, 6. navigate, 7. artificial, 8. minority, 9. degrade, 10. implanted, 11. accident, 12. combination, 13. surgical, 14. miniaturization, 15. electronic, 16. electrode, 17. encapsulate, 18. inch, 19. physiologist, 20. cortex, 21. phosphene, 22. ophthalmologist, 23. seemingly, 24. prostheses, 25. retina, 26. feasible, 27. perch, 28. belt-worn, 29. grid, 30. affix, 31. transmit, 32. distinguish, 33. optic, 34. compression, 35. intermediate, 36. topography, 37. stimulate, 38. theoretically

Exercises 2
(1) F, (2) T, (3) F, (4) T, (5) F

Exercises 3
(1) None of today's devices will work for people who were born blind.
(2) Researchers have investigated the use of electricity to stimulate vision for nearly half a century.
(3) Wireless stimulation of the electrodes made the patient see spots of light known as phosphenes.
(4) The way to stimulate the remaining functional cells was proved feasible in the mid-1990s.
(5) Some of the people could also detect motion when a bar of light was moved in different directions in a darkened room.

Exercises 4
(1) The existing artificial eyes benefit the minority of blind people who suffer from diseases such as retinitis peigmentosa (RP) and macular degeneration that degrade retinal cells but leave some of the retina intact.
(2) The existing artificial eyes cannot help people who were bron blind and whose visual system as a whole remains underdeveloped.
(3) A combination of improved surgical techniques, miniaturization of electronics, and the techniques of encapsulating electronics in the body are introduced.
(4) The ophthalmorlogies suggested that degrade photoreceptor cells still leave large portions of the retina intact even after a patient has become totally blind, and the way to stimulate the remaining functional cells was

proved feasible.

(5) The glasses consisting of a tiny video camera also contains a belt-worn video processing unit and an electronic box. The video processor wirelessly transmits a simplified picture of what the camera images to the box, and then the retinal implant stimulates cells in a pattern roughly reflecting the information.

Chapter 14
Exercises 1
1. obesity, 2. prevalence, 3. malnutrition, 4. infection disease, 5. widespread,
6. discrimination, 7. chronic disease, 8. epidemic, 9. socioeconomic,
10. hardship, 11. afflict, 12. approximately, 13. abdominal, 14. deposit,
15. abdomen, 16. waist-hip ration, 17. metabolic syndrome,
18. diabetes mellitus, 19. stroke, 20. hypertension, 21. colorectal, 22. renal,
23. esophageal, 24. gastric cardia, 25. endometrial, 26. gallbladder,
27. gallstones, 28. gout, 29. prone, 30. epidemiological, 31. heterogeneous,
32. expenditure, 33. psychological, 34. boredom, 35. compensate,
36. deficiency, 37. instruction, 38. refined, 39. substitution, 40. variability,
41. intramuscular, 42. accumulation, 43. adipose tissue, 44. neurohormone,
45. blunt, 46. adiposity, 47. postulated, 48. allometric, 49. cardiopulmonary,
50. postprandial, 51. circulating, 52. bypass, 53. aerobic activity,
54. flexibility, 55. mobility, 56. apt, 57. conquer, 58. denominator,
59. give up easily

Exercises 2
(1) T, (2) F, (3) T, (4) F, (5) T

Exercises 3
(1) Obesity should no longer be regarded simply as a cosmetic problem affecting certain individuals, but an epidemic that threatens global wellbeing.
(2) Many people eat in response to negative emotions such as boredom, sadness, or anger.
(3) Numerous dietary changes contribute to the reduction in chronic disease risk.
(4) As long as the increase in energy expenditure is sufficient, low-intensity endurance exercise is likely to generate beneficial metabolic

effects.

(5) People who exercise are more apt to stay on a diet plan.

Exercises 4

(1) The current measurement of obesity is defined by a body-mass index (BMI), weight divide by square of the height kg/m^2.

(2) Type 2 diabetes mellitus (adult-onset type), insulin resistance, coronary heart disease (CHD) and stroke, high blood pressure (hypertension).

(3) Gene, exercise, food intake, metabolic rates, culture, and environmental factors

(4) The mainstay of treatment for obesity is an energy-limited diet and increased exercise (physical activity).

(5) Skeletal muscle is responsible for a major portion of uptake glucose in the postprandial state, mediated by an increase in circulating levels of insulin.

(6) Explain your opinions.

Chapter 15
Exercises 1

1. aging, 2. emphasize, 3. desire, 4. deserve, 5. dignity, 6. encompass,
7. hospice, 8. distinction, 9. customer-focused, 10. denture, 11. chew,
12. malnutrition, 13. gastrointestinal, 14. diarrhea, 15. food poisoning,
16. excretion, 17. dehydration, 18. disaster, 19. rehabilitative therapy,
20. bedridden, 21. deterioration, 22. fatigue, 23. aggravation, 24. endure,
25. manifest, 26. anxiety, 27. disturbance, 28. prospects, 29. delirium,
30. agitation, 31. sleep disorder, 32. dementia, 33. exacerbation,
34. vital signs, 35. constipation, 36. incontinence, 37. cognitive function,
38. memory disorder, 39. disorientation, 40. hallucination, 41. delusion,
42. aimless wandering, 43. unclean behavior, 44. pica, 45. sanitary,
46. oral hygiene, 47. respiratory infections, 48. cope, 49. cooperative,
50. beneficiary, 51. respite, 52. consideration

Exercises 2

(1) T, (2) F, (3) T, (4) T, (5) F

Exercises 3

(1) We live in a world that changes from moment to moment, a world in

which we grow old, fall ill, and die.
(2) Care for the elderly is a major concern for all who live in an aging society.
(3) It is necessary to evaluate the health of the elderly and provide support to prevent the aggravation of chronic conditions.
(4) An acute change in the living environment within the shelter may cause a transient brain dysfunction.
(5) Elderly care requires time and energy and no one can cope alone with all demands of care.

Exercises 4
(1) Care is provided when someone can no longer independently carry out essential everyday activities like eating, bathing, dressing, etc.
(2) These factors are length of life and respect of life, and quality of life.
(3) There are food, excretions, mental health and decreased mobility.
(4) Assessment of cognitive function includes memory disorder, disorientation, and misjudgment etc.
(5) Explain your own opinions.

Chapter 16
Exercises 1
1. autonomy, 2. preferences, 3. truthfulness, 4. confidentiality,
5. responsibility, 6. conform, 7. allocation, 8. trustworthiness, 9. integrity,
10. abortion, 11. pertain, 12. sanctity, 13. advocacy,
14. organ transplantation, 15. euthanasia, 16. distributive, 17. recipient,
18. alternative, 19. innocent, 20. deontologist, 21. teleologist,
22. omission, 23. compulsory, 24. comprehensive, 25. surrogacy, 26. monk,
27. enlightened, 28. invade, 29. eugenics, 30. comparable, 31. execute,
32. betraying, 33. heroic, 34. sympathetic, 35. quality of life, 36. profound,
37. implication, 38. dilemma

Exercises 2
(1) F, (2) T, (3) F, (4) T, (5) F

Exercises 3
(1) Doctors have duty to respect patients' decisions and protect the patients who do not have autonomy ability.

(2) Euthanasia is the proactive conduct by terminating the life of a person in a painless or minimally painful way in order to stop suffering or other undesired conditions in life.

(3) Medical expenses are very costly and if no medical insurance, a patient is obliged to encumber the costs by itself. However, illness can strike at anytime unpredictably.

(4) Religious ethics has an influence upon both personal opinion and the greater debate over bioethics.

Exercises 4

(1) Bioethics deals with ethical and value issues gained from life science. Life science is directly associated to life and nature science, including medicine, biology, genetics, medical care, and environment etc.

(2) There are *respect for autonomy, non-maleficence (not harming), beneficence (doing good), justice,* and *Trustworthiness*.

(3) From the end of 1960's to the early of 1970's, the key issue is human experimentation

From the end of 1970's to middle of 1980's, key issues are related to "life" and "death."

From the middle of 1980's, key issue is medical economics. Medical economic issues.

(4) While the rapid development of S&T enrich our daily lives, there are also arising some issues associated to ethical, legal, and social issues (ELSI).

(5) Describe your own opinions.

Index

[A]

abdomen	112
abdominal	112
aberration	68
abortion	50, 131
absorption	17
acelullar	88
acute	50
acute toxicity	21
adipose tissue	116
adiposity	116
administer	77
ADRs (side effects)	23
adverse reactions	6
aerobic activity	117
aggravation	123
aging	122
agitation	124
ailment	62, 63
aimless wandering	124
akinesia	62
allele	75, 76
alleviate	1
allogeneic	88
allometric	116
alteration	75
analgesic drug	2
analytical chemistry	22
anemia	1
aneuploid/aneuploidy	68, 69, 71
animal experiments	21
animal protection	38
antagonist	2
antibiotic	25
antibody	36
antiemetic drugs	8
antipyretic drug	2, 8
antiulcerative drugs	8
anus	9
anxiety	124
aorta	70
appetite	7
artificial	106
artificial organ	36
asthma	7
atherosclerosis	62
athlete foot	51
atom	94
atrophy	63
attenuate	1
autoimmunity	83
autonomic nervous system	62
autonomy	129
autosome	70
avian	50, 52

[B]

bedridden	123
bioactive	90
biocompatible	95
bioethics	129
bioinformatics	58
biological decomposition plastic	40
biomaterial	90
blood clotting	76
blood products	40
bradykinesia	62
brain	50

[C]

carbon	94
cardiopulmonary	116
care-takers	64
catechin	1
cellular	88
cephem	2
cerebral cortex	63
cerebrovascular	62
cerebrum	63
chemical mutagens	68, 69
chemotherapy	84
chills	57
chromosome	68, 69, 70
chronic disease	112
chronic toxicity	21
circulating	116
circulation	57
citrus	2
clinical	20
clinically	88
codominant	75
cognition	100
cognitive function	124
cognitive impairment	63

Index

collagen-rich 88
colorectal 113
compliance 7
concomitant 2
confidentiality 130
constipation 124
constriction 70
convention on biological
   diversity (CBD) 32
cortex 106
criteria 19
cultured 90
customer-focused 122
cystic fibrosis 76
cytogenetics 69

【 D 】

degradation 62
degrade 106
dehydration 123
deletion 68, 69, 75
delirium 124
delusion 124
dementia 62, 124
dementious 62
deontologist 132
deposition 63
depression 63
dermatophytosis 51
deterioration 123
deterrent 2
devices 106
diabetes mellitus 113
diabetics 62
diagnosis 101
diagnostics 58, 94
diarrhea 57, 123
differentiation 82
dignity 122
dilemma 137

disorientation 63, 124
dissociate 90
distribution 17
disturbance 124
duplication 68
dynamic 102

【 E 】

echinococcosis 51
Echinocuccus 51
ecological 32
electrode 106
electronics 106
embryonic/embryo
                50, 69, 88
encephalitis 50
endemic 51
endometrial 113
epidemic 112
epidemiological 52, 63, 114
epitope 58
erythrocyte 57
escalate 19
esophageal 113
esophagus 5
ethics 129
eugenics 137
euthanasia 132, 134
evolution 82
exacerbation 124
excretion 17
expiration date 6
explanted 88
explicitly 100
expressed sequence tag
   (EST) 58

【 F 】

fatigue 123
fetus 50

flavonoid 2
food poisoning 123
forecasted 20

【 G 】

gallbladder 113
gallstones 113
gametic/gamete 69, 71
gastric cardia 113
gastrointestinal 123
gene 63
genetic/genetics 68, 69
genetically 88
genetic engineering
   method 77
genome 75, 77
gonadal streak 70
gout 113
gut 50

【 H 】

haemorrhagic 52
hallucination 64, 124
heavy metal 94
hemoglobin 75
hemophilia 76
hepatocyte 57
hereditary/heredity 68
heritable 63
heterogeneous 114
higher plant 34
hospice 122
host 51
hygiene 53
hyperlipidemia 62
hypertension 62, 113
hypnotic drugs 7
hypoglycemia 7
hypophosphatemia 76

Index

[I]

identification	58
immunity	57
immunity fortifier	40
immunization	57
immunologic	88
immunological dysfunction	75
implanted	106
inapparent infection	50
incidence	52
incontinence	124
infection	25, 50, 57
infectious disease	112
inflammation	50
injured	88
injury	50
innocent	133
insertion	75
intellectual property	21
interaction	100
interface	100
intramuscular	116
inversion	68
irradiation	84
irrespective of	7

[L]

label-free	95
laxatives	1
lethal dose	84
liver	51
locus	75

[M]

malaria	57
malnutrition	70, 112, 123
mammalian	50, 51, 84
manifestation	57
marketability	20
matrices	88
maturation	82
meiosis	69, 70
memory disorder	124
metabolic syndrome	112
metabolism	17
microenvironment	83
miniaturization	106
misfolded	96
mitigate	1
mitosis	69
mobilization	83
molecule	75, 94
monk	135
monosomics	69, 70
monosomy	69, 70
mucus	76
multilineage	82
mutation	75

[N]

nanoscale	94
nanotechnology	94
nanotube	94
naringenin	2
naringin	2
nasal	1
National Cancer Institute (NCI)	35
national inventory	33
nausea	1
neurohormones	116
neuron	62, 63, 64
neuro-physiological	63
new drug	19
nocturnal	7
nondisjunction	69, 70
nucleic acid	75
nullisomics	69

[O]

obesity	112
occurrence	63, 75, 77
ophthalmic	6
ophthalmologist	106
oral hygiene	124
organ transplantation	132
osteoporosis	70
outbreak	51

[P]

palpitation	1
parasite	57, 58
patent application	20
pathogen	50
pathological	63
penicillin shock	23
pentasomy	70
persecution mania	64
pest	50
petrochemical	95
pharmaceutical	95
pharmacochemical	6
phosphenes	106
physics	100
physiologist	106
pica	124
plant biotechnology	38
Plasmodium falciparum parasites	57
polyploidization	69
polyploidy	68, 69
possibility	20
postconception	82
postprandial	116
postural instability	62
premature	19
prevalence	112
prevention	51

Index

prioritization	58	schemic heart disease	62	topography	108
probe	94	sedative drug	2	*Toxocara cati*	50
profit distribution	32	self-renewal	82	Toxocarosis	50
profitability	20	senile	62, 63	Toxoplasmosis	50
promoting the health	17	sensation	2	tracer	95
prostheses	106	sickle cell allele	75	tranquilizers	2
protozoa	50	sickle cell anemia	75	transgenic	77
psychological	115	silicon	94	translocation	68, 71
		sleep disorder	124	transplant	88
[Q]		socioeconomic	112	transplantation	83
quality control	22	somatic	77	treatment	88
		somatic cell	84	trisomics	69
[R]		somatic tissues	84	trisomy	69, 70
rabies	50	spatial sense	63	trustworthiness	130
radiation	57	specificity	52	truthfulness	130
reasonability	17	sporozoite	57		
recessive	76	stakeholder	64	**[U]**	
recipient	88	stem cell	88	ulcer	5
regeneration	82	sterile	70	utero (uterus)	70
rehabilitative therapy	123	streamline	19		
rejection	36	stroke	113	**[V]**	
renal	113	subacute toxicity	21	vaccine	40, 57
renovation	19	subset	82	vascular disorders	62
replicate	90	substitution	75	vector	51
respiratory infections	124	superconductor	94	veterinarian	50
resting tremor	62	suppositories	8	vital signs	124
restriction enzyme	75	supreme	17		
retardant	70	surrogacy	134	**[W]**	
retina	108	sustainable development		waist-hip ration	112
revolutionary	88		34		
rheumatoid arthritis	35			**[X]**	
rickets	76	**[T]**		xonobiotics	2
rigidity	62	tannin	1		
		teleologist	132	**[Y]**	
[S]		tentatively	22	yolk sac	82
safety	17	testicular insufficiency	70		
sanctity	132	tetrasomy	70	**[Z]**	
sanitary	124	thalidomide	23	zoonosis	51
sanitation	53	therapy	88		

―― 編著者・著者略歴 ――

渡邉　和男（わたなべ　かずお）
1983 年　神戸大学農学部園芸農学科卒業
1985 年　神戸大学大学院修士課程修了
1988 年　ウィスコンシン大学大学院博士課程修了（遺伝育種学専攻），Ph. D.
1988 年　国際ポテトセンター主任研究員
1991 年　コーネル大学助教授
1996 年　近畿大学助教授，コーネル大学在外特別準教授
　　　　　国際植物遺伝資源研究所（IPGRI）名誉研究員
2001 年　筑波大学教授
2004 年　筑波大学大学院教授
　　　　　現在に至る

渡邊　高志（わたなべ　たかし）
1983 年　帝京大学薬学部薬学科卒業（薬剤師）
1983 年　農林水産省果樹試験場研究員
1984 年　ネパール王国森林土壌保全省薬草局
1988 年　北里大学薬学部助手
1993 年　ブラジル・アマゾン国立湿潤熱帯農牧研究センター
1999 年　博士（薬学）（北里大学）
2004 年　パキスタン・イスラム共和国コハット工科大学　学位・技術審査員
2007 年　北里大学薬学部助教
2007 年　高知県立牧野植物園・資源植物研究センター
　　　　　現在に至る

王　　碧昭（ワン　ピジャオ）
1975 年　国立台湾大学工学部化学工学科卒業
1975 年　国立台湾工業技術研究院聯合工業研究所勤務
1976 年　台湾国際特許法律事務所勤務
1978 年　台湾 Lee & Li 特許法律事務所勤務
1987 年　筑波大学大学院環境科学研究科修士課程修了
1990 年　東京大学大学院工学系研究科博士課程修了（化学工学専攻），工学博士
1990 年　アメリカ・ニューヨーク州立大学微生物免疫研究所研究員
1991 年　ニューヨーク Cold Spring Harbor 研究所研究員
1994 年　筑波大学講師
1999 年　筑波大学助教授
2003 年　筑波大学教授
2004 年　筑波大学大学院教授
　　　　　現在に至る

陳　　佳欣（チン　ジャシン）
2002 年　台湾逢甲大学環境工学科学学科卒業
2004 年　台湾国立成功大学医学部（環境医学研究科毒理学専攻）修士課程修了
2008 年　筑波大学大学院生命環境科学研究科（生命産業科学専攻）博士課程修了
　　　　　博士（生物科学）
2008 年　筑波大学大学院博士研究員
　　　　　現在に至る

英語で学ぶ医科学入門
Introduction to Medical Sciences and Practices
© K. Watanabe, T. Watanabe, P.-C. Wang and C.-H. Chen　2008

2008年5月23日　初版第1刷発行

検印省略	編著者	渡　邉　和　男
	著　者	渡　邊　高　志
		王　　　碧　昭
		陳　　　佳　欣
	発行者	株式会社　コロナ社
		代表者　牛来辰巳
	印刷所	萩原印刷株式会社

112-0011　東京都文京区千石 4-46-10
発行所　株式会社　コロナ社
CORONA PUBLISHING CO., LTD.
Tokyo　Japan
振替 00140-8-14844・電話 (03) 3941-3131 (代)
ホームページ　http://www.coronasha.co.jp

ISBN 978-4-339-07881-7　(高橋)　(製本：愛千製本所)
Printed in Japan

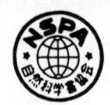

無断複写・転載を禁ずる
落丁・乱丁本はお取替えいたします